THE ULTIMATE CARB CYCLING COOKBOOK FOR BEGINNERS

Carb Cycling Made Simple With 1000 Days of Easy Healthy and Delicious Food Recipes with A New 30-Day Meal Plan and Exercises for Weight Loss - Your Key to A Healthier and Fitter Life

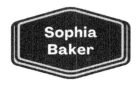

Copyright © 2024 by Sophia Baker

Table of Contents

INTRODUCTION 5

UNDERSTANDING CARB CYCLING 5

PRINCIPLES AND BENEFITS OF CARB CYCLING 5

EXPLORING THE SCIENCE BEHIND CARB CYCLING AND ITS EFFICACY FOR WEIGHT LOSS 5

GETTING STARTED WITH CARB CYCLING 6

NUTRITIONAL FOUNDATIONS OF CARB CYCLING 8

PERSONALIZING CARB CYCLING 9

MAXIMIZING RESULTS WITH PHYSICAL ACTIVITY 11

CHAPTER 1: BREAKFAST RECIPES 14

LOW CARB BREAKFAST 14

1. Veggie and Cheese Omelet 14
2. Avocado Egg Salad 14
3. Keto Chia Seed Pudding 15
4. Greek Yogurt with Berries 15
5. Bacon and Egg Muffins 16
6. Zucchini Hash Browns 16
7. Cauliflower Breakfast Hash 17
8. Almond Flour Pancakes 17
9. Coconut Flour Porridge 18
10. Turkey Sausage Breakfast Skillet 19

HIGH CARB BREAKFAST 19

11. Oatmeal with Fresh Fruit 19
12. Whole Wheat Pancakes with Maple Syrup 20
13. Quinoa Breakfast Bowl 21
14. Sweet Potato Hash with Eggs 21
15. Fruit Salad with Greek Yogurt 22
16. Buckwheat Pancakes with Berries 22
17. Brown Rice Breakfast Bowl 23
18. Multigrain Waffles with Honey 24
19. Blueberry Oat Bran Muffins 24
20. Granola Parfait with Yogurt 25

CHAPTER 2: LUNCH RECIPES 26

LOW CARB LUNCH 26

21. Grilled Chicken Salad with Avocado 26
22. Cauliflower Fried Rice 26
23. Turkey Lettuce Wraps 27
24. Tuna Salad Stuffed Bell Peppers 28
25. Zucchini Noodles with Pesto 28
26. Egg Salad Lettuce Wraps 29
27. Shrimp and Broccoli Stir-Fry 29
28. Greek Salad with Feta and Olives 30
29. Spinach and Mushroom Quiche 31
30. Chicken Caesar Lettuce Wraps 32
31. Salmon Cucumber Roll-Ups 32
32. Keto Eggplant Parmesan 33

33.	Cauliflower Crust Pizza	34
34.	Avocado Tuna Boats	34
35.	Zucchini Lasagna	35

HIGH CARB LUNCH 36

36.	Brown Rice and Black Bean Burrito Bowl	36
37.	Whole Grain Wrap with Hummus and Veggies	37
38.	Sweet Potato and Black Bean Quesadilla	37
39.	Lentil Soup with Whole Grain Bread	38
40.	Pasta Primavera with Whole Wheat Pasta	39
41.	Veggie Sushi Rolls with Brown Rice	40
42.	Falafel Pita Sandwich	40
43.	Couscous Salad with Grilled Vegetables	41
44.	Whole Wheat Pita Pizza	42
45.	Barley and Vegetable Stir-Fry	43
46.	Black Bean and Corn Salad	44
47.	Chickpea and Spinach Curry	44
48.	Whole Grain Pasta Salad with Pesto	45
49.	Lentil and Vegetable Stew	46
50.	Sweet Potato and Kale Salad	47

CHAPTER 3: DINNER RECIPES 48

LOW CARB DINNER 48

51.	Grilled Salmon with Asparagus	48
52.	Chicken Alfredo Zucchini Noodles	48
53.	Beef and Broccoli Stir-Fry	49
54.	Turkey Stuffed Bell Peppers	50
55.	Shrimp and Avocado Salad	51
56.	Smoked Salmon Roll-Ups	51
57.	Eggplant Lasagna Roll-Ups	52
58.	Steak with Garlic Butter Mushrooms	53
59.	Lemon Herb Baked Cod	53
60.	Spaghetti Squash with Meatballs	54
61.	Stuffed Portobello Mushrooms with Spinach and Cheese	55
62.	Chicken and Vegetable Stir-Fry	56
63.	Keto Chicken Parmesan	56
64.	Taco Stuffed Avocados	57
65.	Greek Lemon Chicken Skewers	58

HIGH CARB DINNER 59

66.	Teriyaki Tofu Stir-Fry with Brown Rice	59
67.	Vegetarian Chili with Whole Grain Bread	59
68.	Whole Wheat Pasta with Marinara Sauce	60
69.	Chickpea Curry with Basmati Rice	61
70.	Quinoa Stuffed Bell Peppers	62
71.	Veggie Stir-Fry with Rice Noodles	63
72.	Butternut Squash Risotto	63
73.	Whole Grain Pizza with Vegetables	64
74.	Black Bean Enchiladas with Brown Rice	65
75.	Spinach and Feta Stuffed Peppers with Couscous	66
76.	Lentil and Vegetable Soup with Whole Grain Bread	67
77.	Sweet Potato and Chickpea Buddha Bowl	68
78.	Vegetable Paella	68

79.	Corn and Black Bean Quesadillas	69
80.	Barley Salad with Roasted Vegetables	70

CHAPTER 4: SNACKS AND SMOOTHIES RECIPES 72

Low Carb Snacks 72

81.	Caprese Skewers	72
82.	Stuffed Mini Bell Peppers	72
83.	Cauliflower Hummus	73
84.	Eggplant Chips	74
85.	Cottage Cheese and Tomato Cuts	74
86.	Cucumber and Cream Cheese Bites	75
87.	Stuffed Celery Sticks	75

High Carb Snacks 76

88.	Hummus and Veggie Wrap	76
89.	Fruit and Yogurt Parfait	76
90.	Baked Sweet Potato Fries	77
91.	Banana Nut Muffins	77
92.	Banana Bread	78
93.	Whole Grain Toast with Jam	79
94.	Chocolate Banana Oat Bars	79

Low Carb Smoothies 80

95.	Creamy Vanilla Almond Smoothie	80
96.	Coconut Lime Green Smoothie	80
97.	Coffee Protein Shake	81

High Carb Smoothies 82

98.	Pineapple Coconut Smoothie Bowl	82
99.	Peach Raspberry Smoothie	82
100.	Mango Banana Smoothie Bowl	83

30 DAYS MEAL PLAN 84

CONCLUSION 91

Introduction

Understanding Carb Cycling

Carb cycling is a dietary strategy that revolves around adjusting carbohydrate intake in a cyclical manner. Rather than maintaining a consistent carbohydrate intake every day, individuals alternate between periods of higher and lower carbohydrate consumption throughout the week. Typically, this involves alternating between "high carb" days, where carbohydrate intake is higher, and "low carb" days, where carbohydrate intake is restricted.

The rationale behind carb cycling is rooted in the understanding of how carbohydrates affect insulin levels and metabolic processes in the body. By strategically timing carbohydrate intake, individuals aim to regulate insulin secretion, promote fat burning, and improve metabolic flexibility.

Principles and Benefits of Carb Cycling

The principles of carb cycling revolve around the manipulation of carbohydrate intake to achieve specific metabolic outcomes. The primary principle is to modulate insulin levels by alternating between periods of higher and lower carbohydrate consumption. When carbohydrates are restricted, insulin levels decrease, signaling the body to burn stored fat for energy. On the other hand, when carbohydrates are reintroduced, insulin levels rise, facilitating the uptake of glucose into cells for energy production.

The benefits of carb cycling are multifaceted and extend beyond weight loss. Some of the key advantages include:

1. **Enhanced fat burning:** By cycling carbohydrate intake, individuals can optimize fat metabolism and increase the utilization of stored fat for energy, leading to greater fat loss over time.
2. **Preservation of lean muscle mass:** Unlike traditional calorie-restricted diets, which can lead to muscle loss along with fat loss, carb cycling aims to preserve lean muscle mass by providing adequate protein intake and strategic carbohydrate timing.
3. **Improved metabolic flexibility:** Carb cycling helps the body adapt to efficiently switching between utilizing carbohydrates and fat for fuel, thereby improving metabolic flexibility and resilience.
4. **Sustainable adherence:** Carb cycling offers flexibility and variety in food choices, making it easier for individuals to adhere to their dietary plan long-term compared to more restrictive approaches.
5. **Psychological benefits:** Incorporating higher carbohydrate days can help alleviate feelings of deprivation and promote psychological well-being by allowing for occasional indulgences and treats.

Exploring the Science Behind Carb Cycling and Its Efficacy for Weight Loss

The scientific rationale behind carb cycling lies in its effects on insulin sensitivity, hormone regulation, and metabolic adaptation. Insulin, a hormone synthesized by the pancreas, holds a pivotal role in controlling blood sugar levels and nutrient metabolism. Elevated levels of insulin occur in response to increased carbohydrate intake, prompting the body to store surplus glucose as glycogen in the liver and muscles. However, chronically elevated insulin levels can lead to insulin resistance, a condition characterized by reduced sensitivity to insulin's effects and impaired glucose metabolism.

Carb cycling aims to address this issue by periodically reducing carbohydrate intake, which helps improve insulin sensitivity and promote fat burning. By cycling between high and low carb days, individuals can regulate insulin secretion, prevent metabolic adaptation, and promote fat loss while preserving lean muscle mass.

Furthermore, carb cycling enhances metabolic flexibility, allowing the body to switch between different fuel sources more efficiently. This metabolic adaptability is advantageous for weight loss and overall health, as it enables the body to adapt to fluctuations in dietary intake and energy demands.

Research on the efficacy of carb cycling for weight loss is limited but promising. Some studies have suggested that cycling carbohydrate intake may result in greater fat loss and better preservation of lean muscle mass compared to traditional calorie-restricted diets. Additionally, carb cycling may offer metabolic advantages such as improved insulin sensitivity, enhanced fat oxidation, and increased metabolic rate.

Getting Started with Carb Cycling

Implementing carb cycling effectively requires careful planning, consistency, and adherence to specific guidelines. In this section, we will provide a step-by-step guide to help you get started with carb cycling, tailor the approach to your individual weight loss goals, and offer practical advice for successful implementation.

Step-by-Step Guide to Implementing Carb Cycling

1. **Determine Your Daily Calorie Needs:** Before starting carb cycling, it's essential to calculate your daily calorie requirements based on factors such as age, gender, activity level, weight, height, and weight loss goals. You can utilize online calculators or consult with a nutritionist to determine your calorie needs accurately.

2. **Establish Your Macronutrient Ratios:** Once you have determined your daily calorie target, you need to establish your macronutrient ratios, including carbohydrates, protein, and fat. The exact ratios will depend on your individual goals and preferences, but a common approach for carb cycling is to allocate higher percentages of calories to carbohydrates on high carb days and lower percentages on low carb days.

3. **Set Up Your Carb Cycling Schedule:** Decide on the frequency and timing of your high and low carb days. A typical carb cycling schedule involves alternating between high carb days, moderate carb days, and low carb days throughout the week. For example, you might have three high carb days, two moderate carb days, and two low carb days per week. Alternatively, you could cycle through different carb intake levels on a daily basis.

4. **Plan Your High Carb Days:** During high carbohydrate intake days, prioritize consuming the bulk of your carbohydrates around your workout sessions to enhance performance and aid in recovery. Opt for nutrient-rich complex carbohydrate sources like whole grains, fruits, vegetables, and legumes. Pay attention to portion sizes and steer clear of overindulging in processed or refined carbohydrates

5. **Prepare Your Low Carb Days:** On low carb days, reduce your carbohydrate intake while increasing your intake of protein and healthy fats to compensate for the reduced calories. Emphasize lean

protein options like chicken, turkey, fish, tofu, and legumes, alongside incorporating healthy fats from avocados, nuts, seeds, and olive oil. Ensure to include ample non-starchy vegetables to supply fiber, essential vitamins, and minerals without extraive carbohydrate intake.

6. **Track Your Progress and Make Adjustments Accordingly:** Throughout your carb cycling journey, regularly monitor your progress, including changes in weight, body composition, energy levels, and performance. Monitor your food consumption, exercise regimen, and any shifts in your physical and emotional well-being. Based on your progress and feedback, make adjustments to your carb cycling plan as needed to optimize results and address any challenges or barriers you may encounter. This may involve adjusting your macronutrient ratios, meal timing, or cycling frequency to better align with your goals and preferences.

Tailoring Carb Cycling to Individual Weight Loss Goals

One of the strengths of carb cycling is its flexibility, allowing you to tailor the approach to your specific weight loss goals and preferences. Whether you're looking to lose body fat, maintain muscle mass, or improve athletic performance, carb cycling can be customized to meet your needs. Here are some tips for tailoring carb cycling to your individual weight loss goals:

1. **Fat Loss:** If your primary goal is fat loss, focus on creating a calorie deficit by reducing your overall energy intake while still meeting your protein needs to preserve lean muscle mass. On high carb days, prioritize carbohydrates around your workouts to fuel exercise performance and enhance recovery. On low carb days, emphasize protein and healthy fats to support satiety and promote fat burning.

2. **Muscle Maintenance/Gain:** If you're looking to maintain or gain muscle mass while losing fat, adjust your carb cycling protocol to include more high carb days and prioritize post-workout nutrition. Consume carbohydrates and protein immediately after your workouts to replenish glycogen stores and promote muscle repair and growth. Consider increasing your overall calorie intake mildly to support muscle growth while still maintaining a moderate calorie deficit for fat loss.

3. **Athletic Performance:** If you're an athlete or highly active individual, carb cycling can be an effective strategy for optimizing energy levels and supporting performance. Tailor your carb cycling schedule to coincide with your training schedule, increasing carbohydrate intake around intense workouts or competitions to fuel performance and enhance recovery. Experiment with different carbohydrate sources and timing to find what works best for your individual needs and preferences.

Practical Advice for Successful Carb Cycling

In addition to grasping the principles and mechanics of carb cycling, several practical tips and strategies can aid in your success with this dietary approach:

1. **Plan Your Meals and Snacks**

Take the time to plan and prepare your meals and snacks in advance, especially on low carb days when food choices may be more limited. Stock up on healthy, nutrient-dense foods that align with your carb cycling plan to avoid temptation and impulse eating.

2. **Stay Hydrated**

Drink plenty of water throughout the day to stay hydrated and support overall health and well-being. Aim to consume almost 8-10 glasses of water per day, and more if you're exercising or sweating heavily.

3. **Listen to Your Body**

Pay attention to hunger and satiety cues, and adjust your food intake accordingly. Don't ignore feelings of hunger or deprive yourself extraively on low carb days, as this can lead to overeating or bingeing later on.

4. **Be Flexible**

Be flexible and adaptable with your carb cycling plan, especially when faced with unexpected events or social occasions. Allow yourself to enjoy occasional treats or deviations from your plan without guilt, and get back on track with your next meal or day.

5. **Monitor Your Progress**

Regularly monitor your food intake, energy levels, mood, and progress toward your weight loss objectives. Utilize tools such as food journals, tracking apps, or progress photos to gauge your success and adapt your approach as necessary.

6. **Seek Support**

Enlist the support of friends, family members, or online communities who can provide encouragement, accountability, and guidance throughout your carb cycling journey. Share your goals and progress with others, and celebrate your successes together.

By following these practical tips and strategies, you can increase your chances of success with carb cycling and achieve your weight loss goals in a healthy, sustainable manner. Remember to listen to your body, stay consistent, and be patient as you work towards your desired outcomes.

Nutritional Foundations of Carb Cycling

Achieving success with carb cycling relies heavily on understanding the role of nutrition and making informed food choices. In this section, we will delve into the essential nutritional information for effective carb cycling and discuss how to craft balanced meals that support carb cycling goals.

Essential Nutritional Information for Effective Carb Cycling

To effectively implement carb cycling, it's essential to have a solid understanding of macronutrients and how they impact the body's metabolic processes. Macronutrients include carbohydrates, protein, and fat, each playing a unique role in energy production, muscle repair, and overall health.

Carbohydrates

Carbohydrates serve as the body's primary energy source, vital for supporting both physical and cognitive activities. Upon consumption, they undergo breakdown into glucose, which fuels cellular functions and regulates blood sugar levels. In carb cycling, it's crucial to distinguish between complex carbohydrates, like whole grains, fruits, vegetables, and legumes, and simple carbohydrates, such as refined sugars and processed foods. Complex carbohydrates offer sustained energy and promote feelings of fullness, making them optimal choices for high carb days. Conversely, simple carbohydrates can induce rapid spikes and drops in blood sugar levels, leading to cravings and energy fluctuations, rendering them less suitable for carb cycling.

Protein

Protein constitutes a vital component of any carb cycling regimen due to its role in muscle repair, growth, and maintenance. Sufficient protein intake aids in preserving lean muscle mass, boosting metabolic rate, and promoting satiety, thereby facilitating adherence to a calorie deficit. It's advisable to incorporate lean protein sources such as chicken, turkey, fish, tofu, eggs, or legumes into each meal to bolster your carb cycling objectives.

Fat

Despite its often-misunderstood reputation, dietary fat is an essential macronutrient that plays a variety of critical roles in the body. Fat provides essential fatty acids, supports hormone production, and helps absorb fat-soluble vitamins. Incorporating healthy fats, such as those found in avocados, nuts, seeds, olive oil, and fatty fish, into your diet can help promote overall health and well-being. While fat intake may vary mildly between high and low carb days, it's important to include a moderate amount of healthy fats in your meals to support nutrient absorption and satiety.

Crafting Balanced Meals to Support Carb Cycling Goals

Building balanced meals is essential for optimizing carb cycling results and supporting overall health and well-being. Here's how to craft balanced meals that support your carb cycling goals:

1. **Start with a base of complex carbohydrates:** Choose whole grains, fruits, vegetables, and legumes as the foundation of your meals. These foods provide sustained energy, essential nutrients, and dietary fiber, which promotes satiety and supports digestive health. Aim to fill half of your plate with complex carbohydrates to ensure adequate energy and nutrient intake.

2. **Include a source of lean protein:** Include a serving of lean protein in each meal to support muscle maintenance, repair, and growth. Choose protein sources such as chicken, turkey, fish, tofu, eggs, or legumes and aim to include almost 20-30 grams of protein per meal. Protein-rich foods also help promote satiety and prevent overeating by keeping you feeling full and satisfied between meals.

3. **Incorporate healthy fats:** Incorporate a balanced quantity of healthy fats into your meals to promote overall health and well-being. Choose sources rich in unsaturated fats like avocados, nuts, seeds, olive oil, and fatty fish, as they supply essential fatty acids and contribute to heart health. Adding a serving of healthy fats to your meals can help enhance flavor, promote satiety, and support nutrient absorption.

4. **Include plenty of non-starchy vegetables:** Fill the rest of the portion of your plate with non-starchy vegetables such as leafy greens, broccoli, cauliflower, peppers, and zucchini. These foods are low in calories and high in fiber, vitamins, minerals, and antioxidants, making them ideal choices for supporting weight loss and overall health. Aim to include a variety of colors and textures to maximize nutrient intake and include visual appeal to your meals.

By following these guidelines and crafting balanced meals that include complex carbohydrates, lean protein, healthy fats, and plenty of non-starchy vegetables, you can support your carb cycling goals while enjoying delicious and nutritious meals that nourish your body and support your overall health and well-being.

Personalizing Carb Cycling

While carb cycling holds potential as an effective dietary strategy for numerous individuals, it's crucial to customize the approach to align with your specific needs, preferences, and objectives.

Identifying Suitable Candidates for Carb Cycling

Carb cycling may not be suitable for everyone, and certain factors should be considered when determining if it's the right approach for you. Here are some considerations for identifying suitable candidates for carb cycling:

- **Metabolic rate:** Individuals with a relatively fast metabolic rate may benefit from carb cycling, as the approach can help optimize fat burning and promote weight loss without sacrificing muscle mass. However, individuals with a slower metabolic rate may find it more challenging to achieve significant results with carb cycling and may need to adjust their approach accordingly.

- **Activity level:** Carb cycling can be particularly beneficial for individuals who engage in regular physical activity or have specific performance goals, such as athletes or fitness enthusiasts. By strategically timing carbohydrate intake around workouts, carb cycling can help support energy levels, enhance recovery, and optimize performance.

- **Insulin sensitivity:** Carb cycling might offer particular advantages to individuals dealing with insulin sensitivity problems or metabolic disorders like insulin resistance or type 2 diabetes. By alternating carbohydrate intake and regulating insulin levels, carb cycling could potentially enhance insulin sensitivity and facilitate better management of blood sugar levels.

- **Weight loss goals:** Carb cycling can be an effective strategy for individuals looking to lose body fat while preserving lean muscle mass. However, the approach may not be suitable for individuals with extreme weight loss goals or those with a history of disordered eating. In such cases, it's important to consult with a healthcare professional before starting carb cycling or any other restrictive dietary plan.

- **Dietary preferences and lifestyle:** Carb cycling may not be suitable for individuals who have difficulty adhering to dietary restrictions or prefer a more flexible approach to eating. It's essential to consider your dietary preferences, lifestyle factors, and ability to adhere to a carb cycling plan before embarking on the approach.

Tips for Adapting Carb Cycling to Individual Preferences and Needs

Adapting carb cycling to individual preferences and needs involves customizing the approach to fit your lifestyle, dietary preferences, and goals. Here are some tips for personalizing carb cycling:

1. **Experiment with different cycling frequencies:** There is no one-size-fits-all approach to carb cycling, so experiment with different cycling frequencies to find what works best for you. Some individuals may prefer a more aggressive approach with alternating high and low carb days, while others may benefit from a more moderate approach with fewer fluctuations in carbohydrate intake.

2. **Customize your macronutrient ratios:** Tailor your macronutrient ratios to fit your individual needs and goals. Adjust your protein, carbohydrate, and fat intake based on factors such as activity level, metabolic rate, and dietary preferences. Aim to consume a balance of macronutrients at each meal to support optimal energy levels, satiety, and nutrient intake.

3. **Listen to your body:** Pay attention to how your body responds to carb cycling, including changes in energy levels, hunger and satiety cues, mood, and physical performance. Adjust your carb cycling plan as needed based on your individual feedback and preferences. If you find that certain foods or meal timing strategies work better for you, incorporate them into your carb cycling plan accordingly.

4. **Be flexible:** While it's important to adhere to your carb cycling plan as much as possible, be flexible and adaptable to life's changes and challenges. If you have a special event or social occasion, allow yourself some flexibility in your carb cycling plan and focus on making balanced choices that align with your goals.

By personalizing carb cycling to fit your individual preferences, needs, and goals, you can optimize your results and enjoy long-term success with this flexible and effective dietary approach.

Maximizing Results with Physical Activity

Physical activity stands as a fundamental element of any effective weight loss strategy, including carb cycling. Exercise not only elevates calorie expenditure but also boosts metabolic rate, fosters fat reduction, preserves lean muscle mass, and enhances overall health and wellness.

When combined with carb cycling, physical activity synergistically enhances the effectiveness of the dietary approach by:

- **Increasing calorie expenditure:** Regular exercise increases energy expenditure, helping to create a calorie deficit necessary for weight loss. By burning more calories through physical activity, individuals can achieve a greater calorie deficit, leading to more significant fat loss over time.

- **Enhancing fat burning:** Exercise stimulates lipolysis, the breakdown of stored fat for energy, leading to increased fat burning during both rest and activity. When combined with carb cycling, exercise amplifies the effects of calorie restriction and promotes fat loss while preserving lean muscle mass.

- **Preserving lean muscle mass:** Resistance training and strength exercises help maintain and build lean muscle mass, which is essential for sustaining metabolic rate and achieving a toned, defined physique. By incorporating strength training into your exercise routine, you can preserve muscle mass while losing fat, resulting in improved body composition and overall appearance.

- **Improving metabolic rate:** Regular exercise boosts metabolic rate, the rate at which your body burns calories at rest. By increasing muscle mass, improving insulin sensitivity, and enhancing metabolic efficiency, exercise helps optimize metabolic rate and promote long-term weight maintenance.

- **Enhancing overall health:** Physical activity offers numerous health benefits beyond weight loss, including improved cardiovascular health, enhanced mood and mental well-being, reduced risk of chronic diseases, and increased longevity. By incorporating regular exercise into your lifestyle, you can improve overall health and quality of life while achieving your weight loss goals with carb cycling.

Types of Exercises Beneficial for Weight Loss with Carb Cycling

When it comes to exercise selection, a combination of aerobic and resistance training is ideal for maximizing weight loss and improving body composition with carb cycling. Here are the types of exercises beneficial for weight loss with carb cycling:

1. **Aerobic exercises:** Aerobic or cardiovascular exercises, such as walking, jogging, cycling, swimming, and dancing, are effective for burning calories, improving cardiovascular fitness, and promoting fat loss. Aim to engage in aerobic exercise most days of the week, incorporating both moderate-intensity steady-state cardio and high-intensity interval training (HIIT) to maximize calorie expenditure and fat burning.

2. **Resistance training:** Resistance training, also known as strength training or weightlifting, involves using resistance or weights to build and strengthen muscles. Resistance training helps preserve lean muscle mass, improve metabolic rate, and enhance body composition by increasing muscle definition and tone. Include a variety of resistance exercises targeting major muscle groups, such as squats, deadlifts, push-ups, lunges, and rows, in your workout routine to promote balanced muscle development and strength gains.

3. **High-intensity interval training (HIIT):** HIIT entails alternating between short bursts of intense exercise and brief recovery periods. HIIT workouts are renowned for their efficacy in calorie burning, metabolism boosting, and enhancing cardiovascular fitness within shorter durations compared to steady-state cardio. To optimize calorie expenditure, fat loss, and overall fitness levels, aim to include HIIT workouts in your exercise regimen 2-3 times per week.

4. **Flexibility and mobility exercises:** In addition to aerobic and resistance training, don't forget to integrate mobility and flexibility exercises into your routine to improve joint health, range of motion, and posture. Include activities such as stretching, yoga, Pilates, or mobility drills to maintain flexibility, prevent injury, and enhance recovery between workouts.

5. **Active lifestyle habits:** Aside from dedicated exercise routines, prioritize integrating more movement and physical activity into your everyday life. Opt for the stairs over the elevator, choose walking or biking over driving whenever feasible, and partake in active hobbies or recreational pursuits that bring you joy. Each instance of movement accumulates, contributing to your overall calorie expenditure and success in weight loss endeavors.

Maximizing the Effects of Physical Activity on Carb Cycling Success

To optimize the impact of physical activity on carb cycling success, it's crucial to prioritize consistency, intensity, and progression in your exercise routine. Here are some strategies for maximizing the benefits of physical activity while carb cycling:

1. **Prioritize consistency:** Aim to engage in regular physical activity most days of the week, incorporating a mix of aerobic, resistance, and flexibility exercises to promote overall health and fitness. Schedule your workouts at times that are convenient and sustainable for you, making exercise a non-negotiable part of your daily routine.

2. **Gradually increase intensity:** As your fitness progresses, progressively elevate the intensity and length of your workouts to push your body and sustain advancements toward your weight loss aspirations. Incorporate intervals of higher intensity or heavier weights into your workouts to push your limits and stimulate further adaptations.

3. **Focus on progressive overload:** Incorporate progressive overload principles into your resistance training routine by gradually increasing the weight, reps, or sets of each exercise over time. This will help stimulate muscle growth and adaptation, leading to improvements in strength and body composition. Maintain a workout log to monitor your progress and ensure you're continually challenging yourself.

4. **Listen to your body:** Pay attention to how your body responds to exercise, adjusting the intensity, duration, and frequency as needed to prevent overtraining and promote recovery. Rest and recovery are vital components of any exercise program, so make sure to prioritize sleep, hydration, and proper nutrition to support your body's recovery and repair processes.

5. **Incorporate variety:** Keep your workouts interesting and challenging by incorporating a variety of exercises, workout formats, and training modalities into your routine. This will help prevent boredom, minimize plateaus, and ensure balanced muscle development. Try new activities or classes, experiment with different equipment or training styles, and keep challenging yourself to try new things.

6. **Set realistic goals:** Set specific, measurable, achievable, relevant, and time-bound (SMART) goals for your physical activity and weight loss journey. Whether it's completing a certain number of workouts per week, achieving a new personal best in strength or endurance, or losing a certain amount of weight or body fat, having clear goals can help keep you motivated and focused on your progress.

By prioritizing consistency, intensity, progression, and variety in your exercise routine, you can maximize the effects of physical activity on carb cycling success, leading to greater fat loss, improved body composition, and enhanced overall health and well-being.

Breakfast Recipes

Low Carb Breakfast

1. *Veggie and Cheese Omelet*

Preparation time: 5 minutes

Cooking time: 5 minutes

Servings: 1

Ingredients:

- 2 big eggs
- 1/4 cup chopped bell peppers
- 1/4 cup chopped onions
- 1/4 cup shredded cheese
- Salt and pepper as required

Directions:

1. In your bowl, whisk the eggs 'til well beaten.
2. Warm a non-stick skillet in a middling temp. and coat with cooking spray.
3. Pour the beaten eggs into your skillet.
4. Sprinkle the bell peppers, onions, and cheese uniformly over one half of the omelet.
5. Cook until the bottom is golden brown and the edges are firm, around 3-4 minutes.
6. Over the stuffing, fold the other half of the omelet.
7. Cook for an extra 1-2 minutes 'til the cheese is melted then the omelet is cooked through.
8. Flavour using salt and pepper as required.

Per serving: Calories: 280kcal; Fat: 20g; Carbs: 6g; Protein: 20g; Sugar: 3g; Sodium: 380mg; Potassium: 250mg

2. *Avocado Egg Salad*

Preparation time: 10 minutes

Servings: 2

Ingredients:

- 2 ripe avocados
- 4 hard-boiled eggs, chopped
- 1 tbsp. lemon juice
- Salt and pepper as required

Directions:

1. In your bowl, mash the avocados with a fork 'til smooth.
2. Include the chopped hard-boiled eggs and lemon juice to the mashed avocado.
3. Mix 'til well combined.
4. Flavour using salt and pepper as required.
5. Serve chilled.

Per serving: Calories: 340kcal; Fat: 28g; Carbs: 14g; Protein: 12g; Sugar: 1g; Sodium: 90mg; Potassium: 930mg

3. *Keto Chia Seed Pudding*

Preparation time: 5 minutes (plus chilling time)

Servings: 2

Ingredients:

- 1/4 cup chia seeds
- 1 cup unsweetened almond milk
- 1 tbsp. low-carb sweetener (e.g., erythritol or stevia)
- 1/2 tsp. vanilla extract

Directions:

1. In your bowl, whisk collectively the almond milk, sweetener, and vanilla extract.
2. Stir in the chia seeds 'til well combined.
3. Cover then put in the fridge for almost 2 hours or overnight, 'til the pudding thickens.
4. Stir well prior to presenting and include more almond milk if desired.

Per serving: Calories: 140kcal; Fat: 8g; Carbs: 10g; Protein: 5g; Sugar: 0g; Sodium: 80mg; Potassium: 120mg

4. *Greek Yogurt with Berries*

Preparation time: 5 minutes

Servings: 1

Ingredients:

- 1/2 cup Greek yogurt
- 1/4 cup mixed berries (e.g., strawberries, blueberries, and raspberries)
- 1 tbsp. chopped nuts (e.g., almonds or walnuts)
- 1 tsp. honey or low-carb sweetener (optional)

Directions:

1. Spoon the Greek yogurt into a serving bowl.
2. Top with mixed berries and chopped nuts.
3. Drizzle using honey or sprinkle with low-carb sweetener if desired.
4. Present instantly.

Per serving: Calories: 180kcal; Fat: 8g; Carbs: 15g; Protein: 12g; Sugar: 10g; Sodium: 50mg; Potassium: 200mg

5. Bacon and Egg Muffins

Preparation time: 10 minutes

Cooking time: 20 minutes

Servings: 4

Ingredients:

- 6 big eggs
- 4 slices bacon, cooked and crumbled
- 1/4 cup shredded cheese
- Salt and pepper as required

Directions:

1. Warm up oven to 350 deg. F then grease a muffin tin.
2. In your bowl, whisk the eggs 'til well beaten.
3. Stir in the crumbled bacon, shredded cheese, salt, and pepper.
4. Move the mixture to the muffin tray that has been prepared, filling each cup to the brim around 3/4 full.
5. Bake for 20 minutes or 'til the muffins are set and golden brown.
6. Prior to presenting, let the dish to gently cool down.

Per serving: Calories: 210kcal; Fat: 16g; Carbs: 1g; Protein: 15g; Sugar: 0g; Sodium: 350mg; Potassium: 150mg

6. Zucchini Hash Browns

Preparation time: 15 minutes

Cooking time: 10 minutes

Servings: 2

Ingredients:

- 2 medium zucchinis, grated
- 1 egg
- 2 tbsps. almond flour
- 1/4 tsp. garlic powder
- Salt and pepper as required
- 2 tbsps. olive oil

Directions:

1. Put grated zucchini in your clean kitchen towel and squeeze out extra moisture.
2. In your bowl, whisk the egg.

3. Include the grated zucchini, almond flour, garlic powder, salt, and pepper to the beaten egg. Mix 'til well combined.
4. Warm olive oil in your skillet in a middling temp.
5. Scoop spoonfuls of zucchini mixture into your skillet, pressing down mildly to form patties.
6. Cook for 4-5 minutes on all sides or 'til golden brown and crisp.
7. Take out from the skillet then drain on paper towels.
8. Present warm.

Per serving: Calories: 190kcal; Fat: 15g; Carbs: 8g; Protein: 7g; Sugar: 4g; Sodium: 200mg; Potassium: 450mg

7. Cauliflower Breakfast Hash

Preparation time: 15 minutes

Cooking time: 15 minutes

Servings: 4

Ingredients:

- 4 cups cauliflower florets, chopped
- 1/2 onion, diced
- 1 bell pepper, diced
- 4 slices bacon, chopped
- 2 tbsps. olive oil
- Salt and pepper as required

Directions:
1. Put your cauliflower florets into the blending container and pulse them until they take on a rice-like texture.
2. Warm olive oil in your skillet in a middling temp.
3. Include the diced onion, bell pepper, and chopped bacon to your skillet. Cook 'til vegetables are tender and bacon is crispy.
4. Stir in the cauliflower rice then cook for extra 5-7 minutes, 'til cauliflower is tender.
5. Flavour using salt and pepper as required.
6. Present warm.

Per serving: Calories: 170kcal; Fat: 12g; Carbs: 8g; Protein: 7g; Sugar: 4g; Sodium: 250mg; Potassium: 530mg

8. Almond Flour Pancakes

Preparation time: 10 minutes

Cooking time: 10 minutes

Servings: 2

Ingredients:

- 1 cup almond flour

- 2 big eggs
- 1/4 cup unsweetened almond milk
- 1 tbsp. low-carb sweetener (e.g., erythritol or stevia)
- 1/2 tsp. baking powder
- 1/2 tsp. vanilla extract
- Butter or coconut oil for cooking

Directions:

1. In your bowl, whisk collectively the almond flour, eggs, almond milk, sweetener, baking powder, and vanilla extract 'til smooth.
2. Heat butter or coconut oil in your skillet in a middling temp.
3. Place 1/4 cup of batter onto your skillet for all pancakes.
4. Cook 2-3 minutes on all sides, 'til golden brown.
5. Present warm with the toppings of your choice.

Per serving: Calories: 380kcal; Fat: 30g; Carbs: 10g; Protein: 16g; Sugar: 2g; Sodium: 200mg; Potassium: 180mg

9. *Coconut Flour Porridge*

Preparation time: 5 minutes
Cooking time: 5 minutes
Servings: 1
Ingredients:

- 2 tbsps. coconut flour
- 1/2 cup unsweetened almond milk
- 1/4 tsp. cinnamon
- 1/4 tsp. vanilla extract
- Low-carb sweetener as required
- Optional toppings: cut almonds, shredded coconut, berries

Directions:

1. In your small saucepan, whisk collectively the coconut flour, almond milk, cinnamon, and vanilla extract.
2. Cook in a middling temp., mixing regularly, 'til densed.
3. Sweeten as required with low-carb sweetener.
4. Present warm with optional toppings if desired.

Per serving: Calories: 140kcal; Fat: 5g; Carbs: 15g; Protein: 5g; Sugar: 1g; Sodium: 150mg; Potassium: 150mg

10. Turkey Sausage Breakfast Skillet

Preparation time: 10 minutes

Cooking time: 15 minutes

Servings: 4

Ingredients:

- 1 lb. turkey sausage, casings taken out
- 1 bell pepper, diced
- 1/2 onion, diced
- 2 cups spinach leaves
- 6 big eggs
- Salt and pepper as required

Directions:

1. In your big skillet, cook the turkey sausage in a middling temp. 'til browned then cooked through.
2. Include diced bell pepper and onion to your skillet. Cook 'til vegetables are tender.
3. Stir in the spinach leaves then cook 'til wilted.
4. Crack the eggs into your skillet, uniformly spacing them around the pan.
5. Cover then cook for 5-7 minutes, or 'til eggs are cooked to your taste.
6. Flavour using salt and pepper as required.
7. Present warm.

Per serving: Calories: 320kcal; Fat: 20g; Carbs: 8g; Protein: 26g; Sugar: 3g; Sodium: 750mg; Potassium: 560mg

High Carb Breakfast

11. Oatmeal with Fresh Fruit

Preparation time: 5 minutes

Cooking time: 5 minutes

Servings: 1

Ingredients:

- 1/2 cup rolled oats
- 1 cup milk (any type)
- 1/2 tsp. cinnamon
- 1/2 cup fresh fruit (e.g., berries, cut banana, or chopped apples)
- 1 tbsp. honey or maple syrup (optional)

Directions:

1. In your small saucepan, bring the milk to a simmer in a middling temp.
2. Stir in the rolled oats and cinnamon.
3. Cook 5 minutes, mixing irregularly, 'til the oats are tender then the mixture has densed.
4. Take out from heat then let it sit for a minute.
5. Move the oatmeal to a bowl and top with fresh fruit.
6. In the event that you so prefer, drizzle with honey or maple syrup.

Per serving: Calories: 350kcal; Fat: 7g; Carbs: 60g; Protein: 11g; Sugar: 22g; Sodium: 120mg; Potassium: 450mg

12. *Whole Wheat Pancakes with Maple Syrup*

Preparation time: 10 minutes

Cooking time: 10 minutes

Servings: 2

Ingredients:

- 1 cup whole wheat flour
- 1 tbsp. sugar
- 1 tsp. baking powder
- 1/4 tsp. salt
- 1 cup milk (any type)
- 1 big egg
- 2 tbsps. vegetable oil
- Maple syrup for presenting

Directions:

1. In your big bowl, whisk collectively the whole wheat flour, sugar, baking powder, and salt.
2. In your distinct bowl, whisk collectively the milk, egg, and vegetable oil.
3. Pour the wet components in to your dry components then stir 'til just combined.
4. Warm a non-stick skillet or griddle in a middling temp. then mildly oil with oil or butter.
5. Place 1/4 cup of batter onto your skillet for all pancakes.
6. Cook until bubbles appear on the surface, then flip the food and continue cooking until the other side receives a golden brown color.
7. Present warm with maple syrup.

Per serving: Calories: 380kcal; Fat: 14g; Carbs: 55g; Protein: 11g; Sugar: 12g; Sodium: 470mg; Potassium: 330mg

13. Quinoa Breakfast Bowl

Preparation time: 10 minutes

Cooking time: 15 minutes

Servings: 2

Ingredients:

- 1/2 cup quinoa, rinsed
- 1 cup water or milk (any type)
- 1/2 tsp. cinnamon
- 1/4 tsp. vanilla extract
- 1 tbsp. honey or maple syrup
- 1/4 cup chopped nuts (e.g., almonds or walnuts)
- 1/4 cup fresh fruit (e.g., berries or cut banana)

Directions:

1. In your small saucepan, blend the quinoa and water or milk. Attain a boiling point.
2. Decrease the temp., cover, then simmer for 15 minutes, or 'til the quinoa is tender and the liquid is immersed.
3. Take out from heat then stir in the cinnamon, vanilla extract, and honey or maple syrup.
4. Divide the cooked quinoa into bowls.
5. Top with chopped nuts and fresh fruit.
6. Present warm.

Per serving: Calories: 300kcal; Fat: 10g; Carbs: 45g; Protein: 10g; Sugar: 12g; Sodium: 10mg; Potassium: 360mg

14. Sweet Potato Hash with Eggs

Preparation time: 10 minutes

Cooking time: 20 minutes

Servings: 2

Ingredients:

- 1 big sweet potato, skinned and diced
- 1/2 onion, diced
- 1 bell pepper, diced
- 2 tbsps. olive oil
- Salt and pepper as required
- 4 big eggs

Directions:

1. Warm olive oil in your skillet in a middling temp.

2. Include the diced sweet potato to your skillet then cook for 10 minutes, mixing irregularly, 'til tender.
3. Include diced onion and bell pepper to your skillet. Cook for extra 5 minutes, 'til vegetables are softened.
4. Flavour using salt and pepper as required.
5. After that, divide the hash mixture into four equal parts and crack an egg into all of the wells.
6. Cover the skillet then cook for 5-7 minutes, or 'til the eggs are cooked.
7. Present warm.

Per serving: Calories: 320kcal; Fat: 18g; Carbs: 30g; Protein: 13g; Sugar: 9g; Sodium: 120mg; Potassium: 720mg

15. *Fruit Salad with Greek Yogurt*

Preparation time: 10 minutes

Servings: 2

Ingredients:

- 1 cup mixed fresh fruit (e.g., berries, grapes, pineapple, and melon)
- 1/2 cup plain Greek yogurt
- 1 tbsp. honey or maple syrup
- 1/4 cup chopped nuts (e.g., almonds or walnuts)

Directions:

1. Wash and chop the fresh fruit as needed.
2. In your bowl, blend the mixed fruit and Greek yogurt.
3. Drizzle using honey or maple syrup.
4. Sprinkle with chopped nuts.
5. Toss carefully to blend.
6. Serve chilled.

Per serving: Calories: 250kcal; Fat: 10g; Carbs: 30g; Protein: 12g; Sugar: 20g; Sodium: 50mg; Potassium: 370mg

16. *Buckwheat Pancakes with Berries*

Preparation time: 10 minutes

Cooking time: 10 minutes

Servings: 2

Ingredients:

- 1/2 cup buckwheat flour
- 1/2 tsp. baking powder
- 1/4 tsp. baking soda
- 1/4 tsp. cinnamon

- 1/2 cup milk (any type)
- 1 big egg
- 1 tbsp. honey or maple syrup
- 1/2 cup mixed berries (e.g., strawberries, blueberries, and raspberries)

Directions:

1. In your big bowl, whisk collectively the buckwheat flour, baking powder, baking soda, and cinnamon.
2. In your distinct bowl, whisk collectively the milk, egg, and honey or maple syrup.
3. Pour the wet components in to your dry components then stir 'til just combined.
4. Warm a non-stick skillet or griddle in a middling temp. then mildly oil with oil or butter.
5. Place 1/4 cup of batter onto your skillet for all pancakes.
6. Cook until bubbles appear on the surface, then turn the food and continue cooking until the other side receives a golden brown color.
7. Present warm with mixed berries.

Per serving: Calories: 320kcal; Fat: 6g; Carbs: 60g; Protein: 11g; Sugar: 18g; Sodium: 330mg; Potassium: 490mg

17. Brown Rice Breakfast Bowl

Preparation time: 10 minutes

Cooking time: 20 minutes

Servings: 2

Ingredients:

- 1/2 cup brown rice
- 1 cup water or milk (any type)
- 1/2 tsp. cinnamon
- 1/4 tsp. vanilla extract
- 1 tbsp. honey or maple syrup
- 1/4 cup chopped nuts (e.g., almonds or walnuts)
- 1/4 cup dried fruit (e.g., raisins or cranberries)

Directions:

1. Rinse the brown rice under cold water.
2. In your saucepan, bring the water or milk to a boil.
3. Include the brown rice and decrease temp. to low. Cover then simmer for 20 minutes, or 'til rice is tender and liquid is immersed.
4. Take out from heat then stir in the cinnamon, vanilla extract, honey or maple syrup, chopped nuts, and dried fruit.
5. Divide the rice mixture into bowls and serve warm.

Per serving: Calories: 350kcal; Fat: 10g; Carbs: 60g; Protein: 7g; Sugar: 15g; Sodium: 10mg; Potassium: 230mg

18. Multigrain Waffles with Honey

Preparation time: 10 minutes

Cooking time: 10 minutes

Servings: 2

Ingredients:

- 1 cup multigrain pancake/waffle mix
- 1 big egg
- 1/2 cup milk (any type)
- 2 tbsps. vegetable oil
- Honey for presenting

Directions:

1. Warm up waffle iron as per to the manufacturer's directions.
2. In your bowl, whisk collectively the multigrain pancake/waffle mix, egg, milk, and vegetable oil 'til smooth.
3. Pour batter onto warmed up waffle iron then cook as per to the manufacturer's directions, 'til golden brown and crispy.
4. Present warm with honey drizzled on top.

Per serving: Calories: 380kcal; Fat: 16g; Carbs: 48g; Protein: 10g; Sugar: 12g; Sodium: 480mg; Potassium: 210mg

19. Blueberry Oat Bran Muffins

Preparation time: 15 minutes

Cooking time: 20 minutes

Servings: 12

Ingredients:

- 1 cup oat bran
- 1 cup whole wheat flour
- 1/2 cup brown sugar
- 1 tsp. baking powder
- 1/2 tsp. baking soda
- 1/4 tsp. salt
- 1 cup milk (any type)
- 1/4 cup vegetable oil
- 1 big egg

- 1 cup fresh or frozen blueberries

Directions:

1. Warm up oven to 375 deg.F. Grease or line your muffin tin with liners.
2. In your big bowl, blend collectively baking powder, baking soda, oat bran, whole wheat flour, brown sugar, and salt.
3. In your distinct bowl, whisk collectively milk, vegetable oil, and egg.
4. Place wet components into your dry components then stir 'til just combined. Fold in blueberries.
5. Divide batter uniformly among muffin cups.
6. Place in the oven and bake for 18 to 20 minutes, or until a toothpick should come out undamaged when immersed into the middle.
7. Allow the muffins to cool for a couple of minutes in the tray before moving them to a wire rack to finish cooling entirely.

Per serving: Calories: 180kcal; Fat: 6g; Carbs: 28g; Protein: 4g; Sugar: 11g; Sodium: 150mg; Potassium: 170mg

20. Granola Parfait with Yogurt

Preparation time: 5 minutes

Servings: 1

Ingredients:

- 1/2 cup Greek yogurt
- 1/4 cup granola
- 1/4 cup mixed fresh fruit (e.g., berries, cut banana, or chopped apple)
- 1 tbsp. honey or maple syrup (optional)

Directions:

1. In your serving glass or bowl, layer Greek yogurt, granola, and mixed fresh fruit.
2. In the event that you so prefer, drizzle with honey or maple syrup.
3. Repeat layers if desired.
4. Present instantly.

Per serving: Calories: 320kcal; Fat: 8g; Carbs: 52g; Protein: 16g; Sugar: 28g; Sodium: 150mg; Potassium: 300mg

Lunch Recipes

Low Carb Lunch

21. *Grilled Chicken Salad with Avocado*

Preparation time: 10 minutes

Cooking time: 15 minutes

Servings: 2

Ingredients:

- 2 boneless, skinless chicken breasts
- Salt and pepper as required
- 4 cups mixed salad greens
- 1 avocado, cut
- 1/4 cup cherry tomatoes, divided
- 1/4 cup cucumber, cut
- 2 tbsps. olive oil
- 1 tbsp. balsamic vinegar

Directions:

1. Warm up grill to med-high temp.
2. Flavour chicken breasts using salt and pepper.
3. Grill chicken 6-8 minutes on all sides, or 'til cooked through.
4. Let chicken rest for a couple of minutes, then slice.
5. In your big bowl, blend mixed salad greens, cut avocado, cherry tomatoes, and cucumber.
6. Drizzle using olive oil and balsamic vinegar, then toss to coat.
7. Divide salad between plates and top with cut grilled chicken.

Per serving: Calories: 350kcal; Fat: 22g; Carbs: 11g; Protein: 28g; Sugar: 3g; Sodium: 150mg; Potassium: 950mg

22. *Cauliflower Fried Rice*

Preparation time: 15 minutes

Cooking time: 10 minutes

Servings: 4

Ingredients:

- 1 head cauliflower, grated or riced
- 2 tbsps. sesame oil

- 2 pieces garlic, crushed
- 1/2 onion, diced
- 1 cup mixed vegetables (e.g., peas, carrots, and bell peppers)
- 2 eggs, beaten
- 2 tbsps. soy sauce or tamari
- 2 green onions, cut
- Salt and pepper as required

Directions:

1. In your big skillet or wok, heat sesame oil in a middling temp.
2. Include crushed garlic and diced onion, then cook 'til softened.
3. Stir in mixed vegetables then cook 'til tender.
4. Push vegetables to one side of the skillet and pour beaten eggs into the other side.
5. Scramble eggs 'til cooked through, then mix with vegetables.
6. Include grated cauliflower to your skillet then stir well to blend.
7. Pour soy sauce or tamari over cauliflower mixture then toss 'til uniformly coated.
8. Cook for extra 5-7 minutes, or 'til cauliflower is tender.
9. Flavour using salt and pepper as required, and garnish with cut green onions prior to presenting.

Per serving: Calories: 150kcal; Fat: 9g; Carbs: 12g; Protein: 7g; Sugar: 5g; Sodium: 450mg; Potassium: 620mg

23. *Turkey Lettuce Wraps*

Preparation time: 10 minutes

Cooking time: 10 minutes

Servings: 4

Ingredients:

- 1 lb. ground turkey
- 2 pieces garlic, crushed
- 1 tbsp. ginger, crushed
- 1/4 cup soy sauce or tamari
- 2 tbsps. rice vinegar
- 1 tbsp. sesame oil
- 1 tbsp. Sriracha sauce (optional)
- 1/4 cup green onions, cut
- 1/4 cup chopped peanuts or cashews
- 1 head iceberg or butter lettuce, that is leaves distinctd

Directions:

1. In your big skillet, cook ground turkey in a middling temp. 'til browned then cooked through.
2. Include crushed garlic and ginger to your skillet then cook for extra 1-2 minutes.

3. Stir in soy sauce or tamari, rice vinegar, sesame oil, and Sriracha sauce (if using). Cook for an extra 2-3 minutes.
4. Take out from heat then stir in cut green onions and chopped nuts.
5. Spoon turkey mixture onto lettuce leaves, then roll up to form wraps.
6. Present instantly.

Per serving: Calories: 250kcal; Fat: 15g; Carbs: 6g; Protein: 22g; Sugar: 2g; Sodium: 650mg; Potassium: 380mg

24. Tuna Salad Stuffed Bell Peppers

Preparation time: 10 minutes

Servings: 4

Ingredients:

- 10 oz tuna
- 1/4 cup mayonnaise
- 1 tbsp. Dijon mustard
- 1/4 cup diced celery
- 1/4 cup diced red onion
- Salt and pepper as required
- 4 big bell peppers, divided and seeded
- Optional toppings: cut avocado, chopped parsley

Directions:

1. In your bowl, blend collectively tuna, mayonnaise, Dijon mustard, celery, and red onion.
2. Flavour using salt and pepper as required.
3. Spoon tuna salad mixture into divided bell peppers.
4. Top with optional toppings if desired.
5. Serve chilled or at room temp.

Per serving: Calories: 200kcal; Fat: 9g; Carbs: 9g; Protein: 21g; Sugar: 5g; Sodium: 300mg; Potassium: 650mg

25. Zucchini Noodles with Pesto

Preparation time: 15 minutes

Cooking time: 5 minutes

Servings: 2

Ingredients:

- 2 medium zucchini, spiralized into noodles
- 1/4 cup pesto sauce
- 1/4 cup cherry tomatoes, divided
- 2 tbsps. grated Parmesan cheese

- Salt and pepper as required

Directions:

1. Warm a big skillet in a middling temp.
2. Include spiralized zucchini noodles to your skillet then cook for 2-3 minutes, or 'til just tender.
3. Stir in pesto sauce and cherry tomatoes, then cook for an extra 1-2 minutes, 'til heated through.
4. Take out from heat then flavour using salt and pepper as required.
5. Present warm, sprinkled with grated Parmesan cheese.

Per serving: Calories: 180kcal; Fat: 13g; Carbs: 10g; Protein: 7g; Sugar: 5g; Sodium: 300mg; Potassium: 670mg

26. Egg Salad Lettuce Wraps

Preparation time: 10 minutes

Cooking time: 10 minutes

Servings: 4

Ingredients:

- 6 hard-boiled eggs, chopped
- 1/4 cup mayonnaise
- 1 tbsp. Dijon mustard
- 2 tbsps. chopped fresh dill or parsley
- Salt and pepper as required
- 8 big lettuce leaves (e.g., butter lettuce or romaine)
- Optional toppings: cut avocado, tomato slices

Directions:

1. In your bowl, blend collectively chopped hard-boiled eggs, mayonnaise, Dijon mustard, chopped fresh dill or parsley, salt, and pepper.
2. Lay out lettuce leaves on a flat surface.
3. Spoon egg salad mixture onto each lettuce leaf.
4. Top with optional toppings if desired.
5. Roll up lettuce leaves to form wraps.
6. Present instantly.

Per serving: Calories: 250kcal; Fat: 20g; Carbs: 2g; Protein: 12g; Sugar: 1g; Sodium: 300mg; Potassium: 260mg

27. Shrimp and Broccoli Stir-Fry

Preparation time: 10 minutes

Cooking time: 10 minutes

Servings: 4

Ingredients:

- 1 lb. shrimp, skinned and deveined
- 2 cups broccoli florets
- 2 pieces garlic, crushed
- 1 tbsp. ginger, crushed
- 1/4 cup soy sauce or tamari
- 1 tbsp. sesame oil
- 1 tbsp. olive oil
- 2 green onions, cut
- Sesame seeds for garnish (optional)

Directions:

1. In your big skillet or wok, warm olive oil in a med-high temp.
2. Include crushed garlic and ginger to your skillet then cook 'til fragrant.
3. Include shrimp to your skillet then cook 'til pink and opaque, 2-3 minutes on all sides. Take out shrimp from skillet then put away.
4. In the similar skillet, include broccoli florets then stir-fry for 3-4 minutes, or 'til tender-crisp.
5. Return cooked shrimp to your skillet.
6. Pour soy sauce or tamari and sesame oil over shrimp and broccoli. Stir well to blend.
7. Cook for an extra 1-2 minutes, 'til heated through.
8. Garnish using cut green onions and sesame seeds if desired.

Per serving: Calories: 200kcal; Fat: 8g; Carbs: 7g; Protein: 25g; Sugar: 2g; Sodium: 600mg; Potassium: 420mg

28. Greek Salad with Feta and Olives

Preparation time: 10 minutes

Servings: 2

Ingredients:

- 4 cups mixed salad greens
- 1/2 cucumber, cut
- 1/2 cup cherry tomatoes, divided
- 1/4 cup cut red onion
- 1/4 cup crumbled feta cheese
- 1/4 cup Kalamata olives
- 2 tbsps. olive oil
- 1 tbsp. red wine vinegar
- 1 tsp. dried oregano
- Salt and pepper as required

Directions:

1. In your big bowl, blend mixed cherry tomatoes, salad greens, cut cucumber, and cut red onion.
2. Place crumbled feta cheese and Kalamata olives to the bowl.
3. In your small bowl, whisk collectively salt, olive oil, red wine vinegar, dried oregano, and pepper.
4. Drizzle dressing over salad then toss carefully to blend.
5. Present instantly.

Per serving: Calories: 250kcal; Fat: 20g; Carbs: 10g; Protein: 5g; Sugar: 4g; Sodium: 400mg; Potassium: 400mg

29. *Spinach and Mushroom Quiche*

Preparation time: 15 minutes

Cooking time: 40 minutes

Servings: 6

Ingredients:

- 1 store-bought or homemade pie crust
- 1 tbsp. olive oil
- 1/2 onion, diced
- 2 cups fresh spinach leaves
- 1 cup cut mushrooms
- 4 big eggs
- 1 cup milk (any type)
- 1/2 cup shredded cheese (e.g., cheddar or mozzarella)
- Salt and pepper as required

Directions:

1. Warm up oven to 375 deg.F.
2. Place pie crust in your pie dish and crimp edges as desired.
3. In your skillet, warm olive oil in a middling temp. Include diced onion then cook 'til softened.
4. Include spinach leaves and cut mushrooms to your skillet. Cook 'til spinach is wilted and mushrooms are tender.
5. In your bowl, whisk collectively eggs, milk, shredded cheese, salt, and pepper.
6. Disperse cooked spinach and mushrooms uniformly over the bottom of the pie crust.
7. Pour egg mixture over your spinach and mushrooms.
8. Bake for 35-40 minutes, or 'til quiche is set and golden brown on top.
9. Allow quiche to cool for a couple of minutes prior to cutting and serving.

Per serving: Calories: 300kcal; Fat: 20g; Carbs: 20g; Protein: 12g; Sugar: 4g; Sodium: 300mg; Potassium: 350mg

30. Chicken Caesar Lettuce Wraps

Preparation time: 10 minutes

Cooking time: 15 minutes

Servings: 4

Ingredients:

- 1 lb. boneless, skinless chicken breasts
- Salt and pepper as required
- 2 tbsps. olive oil
- 1/4 cup Caesar dressing
- 1/4 cup grated Parmesan cheese
- 1 head romaine lettuce, leaves distinctd
- Optional toppings: cherry tomatoes, croutons

Directions:

1. Flavour chicken breasts using salt and pepper.
2. Warm olive oil in your skillet in a med-high temp. Include chicken breasts then cook for 6-8 minutes on all sides, or 'til cooked through.
3. Take out chicken from skillet then let it rest for a couple of minutes. Then slice into strips.
4. In your bowl, toss cut chicken with Caesar dressing and grated Parmesan cheese 'til uniformly coated.
5. Lay out romaine lettuce leaves on a flat surface.
6. Spoon chicken mixture onto each lettuce leaf.
7. Top with optional toppings if desired.
8. Present instantly.

Per serving: Calories: 250kcal; Fat: 12g; Carbs: 3g; Protein: 30g; Sugar: 1g; Sodium: 350mg; Potassium: 500mg

31. Salmon Cucumber Roll-Ups

Preparation time: 15 minutes

Servings: 2

Ingredients:

- 4 oz smoked salmon
- 1 cucumber
- 1/4 cup cream cheese
- 1 tbsp. chopped fresh dill
- Salt and pepper as required

Directions:

1. Cut cucumber lengthwise into fine strips using a vegetable peeler or mandoline.

2. Lay out cucumber slices on a flat surface.
3. Put a fine layer of a cream cheese onto each cucumber slice.
4. Put a piece of smoked salmon at one end of each cucumber slice.
5. Sprinkle chopped fresh dill over the salmon.
6. Roll up the cucumber slices firmly to form roll-ups.
7. Secure with toothpicks if necessary.
8. Serve chilled.

Per serving: Calories: 180kcal; Fat: 12g; Carbs: 5g; Protein: 12g; Sugar: 2g; Sodium: 400mg; Potassium: 400mg

32. Keto Eggplant Parmesan

Preparation time: 20 minutes
Cooking time: 40 minutes
Servings: 4
Ingredients:

- 1 big eggplant, cut into rounds
- Salt
- 1 cup almond flour
- 2 big eggs, beaten
- 1 cup marinara sauce
- 1 cup shredded mozzarella cheese
- 1/4 cup grated Parmesan cheese
- Fresh basil leaves for garnish

Directions:

1. Warm up oven to 400 deg.F.
2. Place eggplant slices on your baking sheet lined using paper towels. Sprinkle both sides with salt then let sit for 15 minutes to draw out moisture.
3. Pat eggplant slices dry using paper towels.
4. Set up a breading station with almond flour in one shallow dish and beaten eggs in another.
5. Dip each eggplant slice in to your beaten eggs, then coat with almond flour.
6. Place breaded eggplant slices on a greased baking sheet.
7. Bake in to your warmed up oven for 20 minutes, flipping halfway through, 'til golden brown and crispy.
8. Take out from oven then top each eggplant slice with marinara sauce, shredded mozzarella cheese, and grated Parmesan cheese.
9. Return to the oven then bake for an extra 15-20 minutes, 'til cheese is melted and bubbly.
10. Garnish using fresh basil leaves prior to presenting.

Per serving: Calories: 350kcal; Fat: 22g; Carbs: 14g; Protein: 20g; Sugar: 7g; Sodium: 600mg; Potassium: 550mg

33. Cauliflower Crust Pizza

Preparation time: 20 minutes

Cooking time: 30 minutes

Servings: 4

Ingredients:

- 1 head cauliflower, grated or riced
- 1/2 cup shredded mozzarella cheese
- 1/4 cup grated Parmesan cheese
- 1 tsp. dried oregano
- 1/2 tsp. garlic powder
- 2 big eggs, beaten
- 1/4 cup marinara sauce
- Toppings of your choice (e.g., cut pepperoni, bell peppers, mushrooms, onions)

Directions:

1. Warm up oven to 400 deg.F.
2. Place grated or riced cauliflower in your microwave-safe bowl then microwave on high for 5-6 minutes, 'til softened.
3. Let cauliflower cool, then transfer to a clean kitchen towel and squeeze out extra moisture.
4. In your big bowl, blend cauliflower, shredded mozzarella cheese, grated Parmesan cheese, dried oregano, garlic powder, and beaten eggs. Mix 'til well combined.
5. Line your baking sheet using parchment paper and press cauliflower mixture into a thin crust shape.
6. Bake crust in to your warmed up oven for 20 minutes, 'til golden brown and crisp around the edges.
7. Take out crust from oven and spread marinara sauce uniformly over the top.
8. Include toppings of your choice.
9. Return to the oven then bake for an extra 10 minutes, 'til toppings are heated through.
10. Cut and serve.

Per serving: Calories: 200kcal; Fat: 10g; Carbs: 15g; Protein: 14g; Sugar: 5g; Sodium: 450mg; Potassium: 600mg

34. Avocado Tuna Boats

Preparation time: 10 minutes

Servings: 2

Ingredients:

- 1 ripe avocado

- 5 oz tuna
- 2 tbsps. mayonnaise
- 1 tbsp. Dijon mustard
- 1 tbsp. lemon juice
- Salt and pepper as required
- Optional toppings: chopped fresh parsley, cherry tomatoes

Directions:
1. Cut avocado in half lengthwise then take out the pit.
2. Scoop out some flesh from each of your avocado half to create a huge cavity for filling.
3. In your bowl, blend collectively drained tuna, mayonnaise, Dijon mustard, lemon juice, salt, and pepper.
4. Spoon tuna mixture into the hollowed-out avocado halves.
5. Top with optional toppings if desired.
6. Present instantly.

Per serving: Calories: 300kcal; Fat: 25g; Carbs: 8g; Protein: 15g; Sugar: 1g; Sodium: 300mg; Potassium: 550mg

35. Zucchini Lasagna

Preparation time: 20 minutes
Cooking time: 45 minutes
Servings: 4
Ingredients:

- 2 big zucchini, cut lengthwise into fine strips
- 1 cup marinara sauce
- 1 lb. ground turkey or beef
- 1/2 onion, diced
- 2 pieces garlic, crushed
- 1 tsp. dried oregano
- 1 tsp. dried basil
- 1 cup ricotta cheese
- 1 cup shredded mozzarella cheese
- Salt and pepper as required
- Fresh basil leaves for garnish

Directions:
1. Warm up oven to 375 deg.F.
2. In your skillet, cook ground turkey or beef in a middling temp. 'til browned. Drain extra fat.
3. Place diced onion and crushed garlic to your skillet then cook 'til softened.

4. Stir in dried oregano and dried basil. Flavour using salt and pepper as required.
5. Put a fine layer of marinara sauce in the bottom of a baking dish.
6. Organize a layer of your zucchini slices over the marinara sauce.
7. Disperse half of the cooked meat mixture over the zucchini slices.
8. Dollop half of the ricotta cheese over the meat mixture.
9. Sprinkle using half of the shredded mozzarella cheese.
10. Repeat layers using the rest of the components, ending with a layer of zucchini slices on top.
11. Cover baking dish using foil then bake in to your warmed up oven for 30 minutes.
12. Take out foil then bake for extra 15 minutes, 'til lasagna is bubbly and cheese is melted and golden brown.
13. Let lasagna cool for a couple of minutes prior to cutting.
14. Garnish using fresh basil leaves prior to presenting.

Per serving: Calories: 350kcal; Fat: 20g; Carbs: 10g; Protein: 30g; Sugar: 6g; Sodium: 600mg; Potassium: 750mg

High Carb Lunch

36. Brown Rice and Black Bean Burrito Bowl

Preparation time: 10 minutes

Cooking time: 20 minutes

Servings: 2

Ingredients:

- 1 cup cooked brown rice
- 1 cup black beans
- 1 cup diced tomatoes
- 1/2 cup corn kernels
- 1/4 cup diced red onion
- 1/4 cup chopped fresh cilantro
- 1 avocado, cut
- Juice of 1 lime
- Salt and pepper as required

Directions:

1. In your bowl, blend cooked brown rice, black beans, diced tomatoes, corn kernels, diced red onion, and chopped fresh cilantro.
2. Squeeze lime juice over the mixture then toss to blend.
3. Flavour using salt and pepper as required.

4. Divide the burrito bowl mixture between two bowls.
5. Top with cut avocado.

Per serving: Calories: 400kcal; Fat: 18g; Carbs: 55g; Protein: 12g; Sugar: 5g; Sodium: 300mg; Potassium: 800mg

37. Whole Grain Wrap with Hummus and Veggies

Preparation time: 10 minutes

Servings: 1

Ingredients:

- 1 whole grain wrap
- 2 tbsps. hummus
- 1/4 cup shredded carrots
- 1/4 cup cut cucumber
- 1/4 cup baby spinach leaves
- 1/4 cup cut bell peppers
- Salt and pepper as required

Directions:
1. Lay out the whole grain wrap on a flat surface.
2. Disperse hummus uniformly over the wrap.
3. Organize shredded carrots, cut cucumber, baby spinach leaves, and cut bell peppers on top of the hummus.
4. Flavour using salt and pepper as required.
5. Roll up the wrap firmly.
6. Cut in half if desired, and serve.

Per serving: Calories: 300kcal; Fat: 8g; Carbs: 45g; Protein: 10g; Sugar: 6g; Sodium: 600mg; Potassium: 400mg

38. Sweet Potato and Black Bean Quesadilla

Preparation time: 15 minutes

Cooking time: 15 minutes

Servings: 2

Ingredients:

- 2 big whole wheat tortillas
- 1 cup mashed sweet potato
- 1 cup black beans
- 1/2 cup shredded cheddar cheese
- 1/4 cup chopped fresh cilantro

- 1/4 cup diced red onion
- 1 tsp. ground cumin
- 1/2 tsp. chili powder
- Salt and pepper as required
- Olive oil for cooking

Directions:

1. In your bowl, blend collectively mashed sweet potato, black beans, shredded cheddar cheese, chopped fresh cilantro, diced red onion, ground cumin, chili powder, salt, and pepper.
2. Divide the mixture uniformly between two whole wheat tortillas, spreading it over one half of each tortilla.
3. Fold the other half of each tortilla over the filling to create a half-moon shape.
4. Warm a big skillet in a middling temp. and mildly brush with olive oil.
5. Place the quesadillas in the skillet then cook for 3-4 minutes on all sides, or 'til golden brown and crispy.
6. Take out from skillet then let cool for a couple of minutes prior to cutting.
7. Present warm, with salsa or Greek yogurt for soaking if desired.

Per serving: Calories: 450kcal; Fat: 12g; Carbs: 65g; Protein: 18g; Sugar: 8g; Sodium: 700mg; Potassium: 800mg

39. Lentil Soup with Whole Grain Bread

Preparation time: 15 minutes

Cooking time: 30 minutes

Servings: 4

Ingredients:

- 1 cup dried lentils
- 4 cups vegetable broth
- 1 onion, diced
- 2 carrots, diced
- 2 celery stalks, diced
- 2 pieces garlic, crushed
- 1 tsp. dried thyme
- 1 bay leaf
- Salt and pepper as required
- Chopped fresh parsley for garnish
- Whole grain bread for presenting

Directions:

1. Rinse dried lentils under cold water then drain.

2. In your big pot, blend lentils, vegetable broth, diced onion, diced carrots, diced celery, crushed garlic, dried thyme, and bay leaf.
3. Bring soup to a boil in a med-high temp., then decrease temp. to low then simmer for 25-30 minutes, or 'til lentils and vegetables are tender.
4. Flavour using salt and pepper as required.
5. Take out bay leaf prior to presenting.
6. Ladle soup into bowls, garnish using chopped fresh parsley, and serve with whole grain bread on the side.

Per serving: Calories: 300kcal; Fat: 2g; Carbs: 55g; Protein: 18g; Sugar: 8g; Sodium: 800mg; Potassium: 900mg

40. *Pasta Primavera with Whole Wheat Pasta*

Preparation time: 15 minutes

Cooking time: 15 minutes

Servings: 4

Ingredients:

- 8 oz whole wheat pasta
- 2 tbsps. olive oil
- 2 pieces garlic, crushed
- 1 onion, finely cut
- 2 carrots, julienned
- 1 bell pepper, finely cut
- 1 cup broccoli florets
- 1 cup cherry tomatoes, divided
- 1/4 cup chopped fresh basil
- 1/4 cup grated Parmesan cheese
- Salt and pepper as required

Directions:

1. Cook whole wheat pasta using the package guidelines. Drain then put away.
2. In your big skillet, warm olive oil in a middling temp.
3. Include crushed garlic and finely cut onion to your skillet. Cook 'til onion is softened.
4. Include julienned carrots, finely cut bell pepper, and broccoli florets to your skillet. Cook for 5-6 minutes, or 'til vegetables are tender-crisp.
5. Stir in divided cherry tomatoes then cooked whole wheat pasta. Cook for an extra 2-3 minutes, 'til heated through.
6. Take out skillet from heat then stir in your chopped fresh basil and grated Parmesan cheese.
7. Flavour using salt and pepper as required.
8. Present warm, garnished using additional Parmesan cheese if desired.

Per serving: Calories: 350kcal; Fat: 8g; Carbs: 60g; Protein: 12g; Sugar: 8g; Sodium: 200mg; Potassium: 600mg

41. Veggie Sushi Rolls with Brown Rice

Preparation time: 30 minutes

Cooking time: 20 minutes

Servings: 4

Ingredients:

- 2 cups cooked brown rice
- 4 nori seaweed sheets
- 1 cucumber, julienned
- 1 carrot, julienned
- 1 bell pepper, julienned
- 1 avocado, cut
- Pickled ginger and wasabi for presenting
- Soy sauce or tamari for soaking

Directions:

1. Put a nori seaweed sheet shiny side down on a bamboo sushi mat or clean kitchen towel.
2. Disperse a fine layer of cooked brown rice uniformly over your nori sheet, leaving about 1 inch of space at the top edge.
3. Organize julienned cucumber, carrot, bell pepper, and cut avocado in a line across the center of the rice.
4. Using the bamboo sushi mat or kitchen towel, firmly roll up the nori sheet, starting from the bottom edge.
5. Moisten top edge of the nori sheet with a little water to seal the roll.
6. Repeat with rest of the nori sheets and filling components.
7. Using sharp knife to slice each sushi roll into 6-8 pieces.
8. Serve sushi rolls with pickled ginger, wasabi, and soy sauce or tamari for soaking.

Per serving: Calories: 250kcal; Fat: 5g; Carbs: 50g; Protein: 5g; Sugar: 5g; Sodium: 400mg; Potassium: 600mg

42. Falafel Pita Sandwich

Preparation time: 20 minutes

Cooking time: 15 minutes

Servings: 4

Ingredients:

- 8 falafel balls
- 4 whole wheat pitas

- 1 cup shredded lettuce
- 1 cucumber, finely cut
- 1 tomato, finely cut
- 1/4 cup cut red onion
- Tzatziki sauce or hummus for presenting

Directions:

1. Cook falafel balls using the package guidelines if using store-bought, or prepare homemade falafel.
2. Warm whole wheat pitas in a toaster or microwave 'til heated through.
3. Cut each pita in half to form pockets.
4. Stuff each pita half with shredded lettuce, finely cut cucumber, tomato, and red onion.
5. Place 2 falafel balls into each pita pocket.
6. Drizzle using tzatziki sauce or spread with hummus prior to presenting.

Per serving: Calories: 300kcal; Fat: 10g; Carbs: 45g; Protein: 12g; Sugar: 5g; Sodium: 600mg; Potassium: 400mg

43. Couscous Salad with Grilled Vegetables

Preparation time: 20 minutes

Cooking time: 15 minutes

Servings: 4

Ingredients:

- 1 cup couscous
- 1 1/4 cups vegetable broth
- 1 red bell pepper, cut
- 1 yellow bell pepper, cut
- 1 zucchini, cut
- 1 yellow squash, cut
- 1/4 cup chopped fresh parsley
- 2 tbsps. olive oil
- 2 tbsps. balsamic vinegar
- Salt and pepper as required

Directions:

1. In your medium saucepan, bring vegetable broth to a boil.
2. Stir in your couscous, cover, then take out from temp.. Let couscous steam for 5 minutes, then fluff with a fork.
3. In the meantime, heat a grill or grill pan in a med-high temp.
4. In your bowl, toss cut red bell pepper, yellow bell pepper, zucchini, and yellow squash with olive oil, balsamic vinegar, salt, and pepper.

5. Grill vegetables 3-4 minutes on all sides, or 'til tender and mildly charred.
6. In your big bowl, blend cooked couscous, grilled vegetables, and chopped fresh parsley.
7. Toss to blend then adjust seasoning if necessary.
8. Present warm or at room temp.

Per serving: Calories: 250kcal; Fat: 6g; Carbs: 45g; Protein: 8g; Sugar: 5g; Sodium: 400mg; Potassium: 600mg

44. Whole Wheat Pita Pizza

Preparation time: 15 minutes

Cooking time: 10 minutes

Servings: 2

Ingredients:

- 2 whole wheat pita bread rounds
- 1/2 cup marinara sauce
- 1/2 cup shredded mozzarella cheese
- 1/4 cup cut mushrooms
- 1/4 cup cut bell peppers
- 1/4 cup cut olives
- 1/4 cup cut cherry tomatoes
- 1/4 tsp. dried oregano
- 1/4 tsp. dried basil
- Salt and pepper as required

Directions:

1. Warm up oven to 425 deg.F.
2. Place whole wheat pita bread rounds on your baking sheet lined using parchment paper.
3. Disperse marinara sauce uniformly over each pita bread round.
4. Sprinkle your shredded mozzarella cheese over the marinara sauce.
5. Organize cut mushrooms, bell peppers, olives, and cherry tomatoes on top of the cheese.
6. Sprinkle your dried oregano and dried basil over the toppings.
7. Flavour using salt and pepper as required.
8. Bake in to your warmed up oven for 8-10 minutes, or 'til your cheese is melted and bubbly and edges of pita bread are crispy.
9. Take out from oven then let cool for a couple of minutes prior to cutting.
10. Present warm.

Per serving: Calories: 350kcal; Fat: 12g; Carbs: 50g; Protein: 15g; Sugar: 5g; Sodium: 600mg; Potassium: 400mg

45. Barley and Vegetable Stir-Fry

Preparation time: 15 minutes

Cooking time: 20 minutes

Servings: 4

Ingredients:

- 1 cup pearl barley
- 2 cups vegetable broth
- 2 tbsps. vegetable oil
- 1 onion, cut
- 2 carrots, julienned
- 1 bell pepper, cut
- 1 zucchini, cut
- 1 cup snow peas
- 2 pieces garlic, crushed
- 1 tbsp. soy sauce or tamari
- 1 tbsp. hoisin sauce
- Salt and pepper as required
- Sesame seeds for garnish (optional)

Directions:

1. In your medium saucepan, bring vegetable broth to a boil.
2. Stir in pearl barley, cover, and decrease temp. to low. Simmer for 30-40 minutes, or 'til barley is tender and liquid is immersed.
3. In the meantime, heat vegetable oil in your big skillet or wok in a med-high temp.
4. Include cut onion, julienned carrots, cut bell pepper, and cut zucchini to your skillet. Stir-fry for 4-5 minutes, or 'til vegetables are tender-crisp.
5. Include snow peas and crushed garlic to your skillet. Stir-fry for an extra 2 minutes.
6. Stir in cooked pearl barley, soy sauce or tamari, and hoisin sauce. Cook for extra 2 minutes, mixing regularly.
7. Flavour using salt and pepper as required.
8. Garnish using sesame seeds if desired prior to presenting.

Per serving: Calories: 300kcal; Fat: 8g; Carbs: 50g; Protein: 10g; Sugar: 5g; Sodium: 600mg; Potassium: 500mg

46. Black Bean and Corn Salad

Preparation time: 15 minutes

Servings: 4

Ingredients:

- 15 oz black beans
- 1 cup corn kernels
- 1 red bell pepper, diced
- 1/4 cup chopped red onion
- 1/4 cup chopped fresh cilantro
- Juice of 1 lime
- 2 tbsps. olive oil
- 1 tsp. ground cumin
- Salt and pepper as required

Directions:

1. In your big bowl, blend black beans, corn kernels, diced red bell pepper, chopped red onion, and chopped fresh cilantro.
2. In your small bowl, whisk collectively lime juice, olive oil, ground cumin, salt, and pepper.
3. Place dressing over the salad then toss to blend.
4. Adjust seasoning if necessary.
5. Serve chilled or at room temp.

Per serving: Calories: 250kcal; Fat: 8g; Carbs: 40g; Protein: 10g; Sugar: 5g; Sodium: 300mg; Potassium: 700mg

47. Chickpea and Spinach Curry

Preparation time: 15 minutes

Cooking time: 20 minutes

Servings: 4

Ingredients:

- 1 tbsp. vegetable oil
- 1 onion, diced
- 2 pieces garlic, crushed
- 1 tbsp. grated ginger
- 1 tbsp. curry powder
- 1 tsp. ground cumin
- 1 tsp. ground coriander
- 1/2 tsp. turmeric

- 15 oz chickpeas
- 14 oz diced tomatoes
- 1 cup coconut milk
- 2 cups fresh spinach leaves
- Salt and pepper as required

Directions:

1. Heat vegetable oil in your big skillet in a middling temp.
2. Include diced onion to your skillet then cook 'til softened.
3. Stir in crushed garlic, grated ginger, curry powder, ground cumin, ground coriander, and turmeric. Cook for 1-2 minutes, 'til fragrant.
4. Include drained and rinsed chickpeas to your skillet then stir to coat with the spices.
5. Pour diced tomatoes and coconut milk into your skillet. Bring to a simmer.
6. Cook for 10-15 minutes, mixing irregularly, 'til the sauce has densed mildly.
7. Stir in fresh spinach leaves then cook for extra 2-3 minutes, 'til spinach is wilted.
8. Flavour using salt and pepper as required.
9. Present warm, with rice or naan bread if desired.

Per serving: Calories: 300kcal; Fat: 15g; Carbs: 35g; Protein: 10g; Sugar: 5g; Sodium: 500mg; Potassium: 700mg

48. Whole Grain Pasta Salad with Pesto

Preparation time: 15 minutes

Cooking time: 10 minutes

Servings: 4

Ingredients:

- 8 oz whole grain pasta
- 1/2 cup prepared pesto sauce
- 1 cup cherry tomatoes, divided
- 1/2 cup cut black olives
- 1/4 cup pine nuts, toasted
- 1/4 cup grated Parmesan cheese
- Salt and pepper as required

Directions:

1. Cook whole grain pasta using the package guidelines. Drain and wash with cold water.
2. In your big bowl, blend cooked pasta, prepared pesto sauce, divided cherry tomatoes, cut black olives, and toasted pine nuts.
3. Toss to coat the pasta uniformly using the pesto sauce.
4. Sprinkle grated Parmesan cheese over your salad then toss again.

5. Flavour using salt and pepper as required.
6. Serve chilled or at room temp.

Per serving: Calories: 350kcal; Fat: 18g; Carbs: 40g; Protein: 10g; Sugar: 5g; Sodium: 400mg; Potassium: 300mg

49. Lentil and Vegetable Stew

Preparation time: 20 minutes
Cooking time: 40 minutes
Servings: 6
Ingredients:

- 1 cup dried green lentils
- 4 cups vegetable broth
- 1 onion, diced
- 2 carrots, diced
- 2 celery stalks, diced
- 2 pieces garlic, crushed
- 14 oz diced tomatoes
- 1 tsp. dried thyme
- 1 tsp. dried rosemary
- Salt and pepper as required
- Chopped fresh parsley for garnish

Directions:

1. Rinse dried green lentils under cold water then drain.
2. In your big pot, blend green lentils, vegetable broth, diced onion, diced carrots, diced celery, crushed garlic, diced tomatoes, dried thyme, and dried rosemary.
3. Bring stew to a boil in a med-high temp., then decrease temp. to low then simmer for 30-40 minutes, or 'til lentils and vegetables are tender.
4. Flavour using salt and pepper as required.
5. Ladle stew into bowls, garnish with chopped fresh parsley, and serve hot.

Per serving: Calories: 250kcal; Fat: 2g; Carbs: 45g; Protein: 15g; Sugar: 5g; Sodium: 700mg; Potassium: 900mg

50. Sweet Potato and Kale Salad

Preparation time: 20 minutes

Cooking time: 25 minutes

Servings: 4

Ingredients:

- 2 big sweet potatoes, skinned and diced
- 1 tbsp. olive oil
- Salt and pepper as required
- 6 cups chopped kale leaves
- 1/4 cup dried cranberries
- 1/4 cup chopped pecans, toasted
- 1/4 cup crumbled feta cheese
- 2 tbsps. balsamic vinegar
- 1 tbsp. maple syrup

Directions:

1. Warm up oven to 400 deg.F.
2. Place diced sweet potatoes on your baking sheet lined using parchment paper.
3. Pour olive oil over the sweet potatoes then toss to coat. Flavour using salt and pepper.
4. Roast sweet potatoes in to your warmed up oven for 20-25 minutes, or 'til tender and mildly browned.
5. In your big bowl, massage chopped kale leaves with balsamic vinegar and maple syrup 'til mildly wilted.
6. Include roasted sweet potatoes, dried cranberries, toasted chopped pecans, and crumbled feta cheese to your bowl.
7. Toss to blend all components uniformly.
8. Serve chilled or at room temp.

Per serving: Calories: 300kcal; Fat: 10g; Carbs: 45g; Protein: 10g; Sugar: 10g; Sodium: 300mg; Potassium: 900mg

Dinner Recipes

Low Carb Dinner

51. Grilled Salmon with Asparagus

Preparation time: 10 minutes

Cooking time: 15 minutes

Servings: 2

Ingredients:

- 2 salmon fillets
- 1 bunch asparagus, trimmed
- 2 tbsps. olive oil
- 2 pieces garlic, crushed
- Salt and pepper as required
- Lemon wedges for presenting

Directions:

1. Warm up grill to med-high temp.
2. Rub salmon fillets and asparagus with olive oil and crushed garlic.
3. Flavour using salt and pepper.
4. Place salmon fillets and asparagus on the grill.
5. Grill salmon for 4-5 minutes on all sides, or 'til fish flakes simply with a fork.
6. Grill asparagus for 3-4 minutes, turning occasionally, 'til tender-crisp.
7. Take out salmon and asparagus from the grill.
8. Present warm with lemon wedges.

Per serving: Calories: 350kcal; Fat: 20g; Carbs: 6g; Protein: 35g; Sugar: 2g; Sodium: 300mg; Potassium: 900mg

52. Chicken Alfredo Zucchini Noodles

Preparation time: 15 minutes

Cooking time: 15 minutes

Servings: 2

Ingredients:

- 2 medium zucchinis, spiralized into noodles
- 2 boneless, skinless chicken breasts, bite-sized pieces
- 2 tbsps. butter

- 2 pieces garlic, crushed
- 1 cup heavy cream
- 1/2 cup grated Parmesan cheese
- Salt and pepper as required
- Chopped fresh parsley for garnish

Directions:

1. Heat butter in your big skillet in a middling temp.
2. Include crushed garlic to your skillet then cook 'til fragrant.
3. Include chicken breast pieces to your skillet then cook 'til browned then cooked through.
4. Take out chicken from your skillet then put away.
5. In same skillet, include heavy cream and grated Parmesan cheese. Stir 'til cheese is melted and sauce is smooth.
6. Flavour using salt and pepper as required.
7. Include spiralized zucchini noodles to your skillet then toss to coat in the Alfredo sauce.
8. Cook for 2-3 minutes, 'til zucchini noodles are tender.
9. Return cooked chicken to your skillet then toss to blend.
10. Take out from heat then garnish with chopped fresh parsley prior to presenting.

Per serving: Calories: 400kcal; Fat: 25g; Carbs: 8g; Protein: 35g; Sugar: 5g; Sodium: 400mg; Potassium: 800mg

53. Beef and Broccoli Stir-Fry

Preparation time: 10 minutes

Cooking time: 15 minutes

Servings: 2

Ingredients:

- 1/2 lb. flank steak, finely cut
- 2 cups broccoli florets
- 2 tbsps. soy sauce
- 1 tbsp. oyster sauce
- 1 tbsp. sesame oil
- 2 pieces garlic, crushed
- 1 tsp. grated ginger
- 1 tbsp. olive oil
- Sesame seeds for garnish

Directions:

1. In your bowl, marinate finely cut flank steak with soy sauce, oyster sauce, crushed garlic, and grated ginger for 10 minutes.

2. Warm olive oil in your big skillet or wok at high temp.
3. Include marinated flank steak to your skillet then stir-fry for 2-3 minutes, 'til browned.
4. Include broccoli florets to your skillet then stir-fry for an extra 2-3 minutes, 'til tender-crisp.
5. Drizzle sesame oil over the beef and broccoli stir-fry then toss to blend.
6. Cook for extra minute, then take out from temp..
7. Garnish using sesame seeds prior to presenting.

Per serving: Calories: 350kcal; Fat: 20g; Carbs: 10g; Protein: 30g; Sugar: 3g; Sodium: 800mg; Potassium: 900mg

54. Turkey Stuffed Bell Peppers

Preparation time: 20 minutes

Cooking time: 45 minutes

Servings: 4

Ingredients:

- 4 big bell peppers, divided and seeds taken out
- 1 lb. ground turkey
- 1 onion, diced
- 2 pieces garlic, crushed
- 1 cup cooked quinoa
- 1 cup marinara sauce
- 1/2 cup shredded mozzarella cheese
- Salt and pepper as required
- Chopped fresh parsley for garnish

Directions:

1. Warm up oven to 375 deg.F.
2. Place divided bell peppers in your baking dish, cut side up.
3. In your skillet, cook ground turkey, diced onion, and crushed garlic 'til turkey is browned then cooked through.
4. Stir in cooked quinoa and marinara sauce. Flavour using salt and pepper as required.
5. Spoon turkey-quinoa mixture into each bell pepper half.
6. Cover baking dish using foil then bake in to your warmed up oven for 30-35 minutes.
7. Take out foil, sprinkle shredded mozzarella cheese over the stuffed peppers, then bake for extra 10 minutes, or 'til the cheese is melted and bubbly.
8. Garnish using chopped fresh parsley prior to presenting.

Per serving: Calories: 300kcal; Fat: 10g; Carbs: 20g; Protein: 25g; Sugar: 5g; Sodium: 600mg; Potassium: 800mg

55. Shrimp and Avocado Salad

Preparation time: 15 minutes

Cooking time: 5 minutes

Servings: 2

Ingredients:

- 1 lb. shrimp, skinned and deveined
- 2 avocados, diced
- 1 cup cherry tomatoes, divided
- 1/4 cup red onion, finely cut
- 2 tbsps. chopped fresh cilantro
- Juice of 1 lime
- 2 tbsps. olive oil
- Salt and pepper as required

Directions:

1. In your big skillet, warm olive oil in a med-high temp.
2. Include shrimp to your skillet then cook for 2-3 minutes on all sides, 'til pink and opaque.
3. Take out shrimp from the skillet then let cool mildly.
4. In your big bowl, blend finely cut red onion, diced avocado, divided cherry tomatoes, and chopped fresh cilantro.
5. Include cooked shrimp to the bowl.
6. Drizzle your lime juice and olive oil over the salad.
7. Flavour using salt and pepper as required.
8. Toss carefully to blend all components.
9. Serve chilled or at room temp.

Per serving: Calories: 350kcal; Fat: 20g; Carbs: 15g; Protein: 30g; Sugar: 5g; Sodium: 400mg; Potassium: 900mg

56. Smoked Salmon Roll-Ups

Preparation time: 10 minutes

Servings: 2

Ingredients:

- 4 slices smoked salmon
- 4 tbsps. cream cheese
- 1 tbsp. chopped chives

Directions:

1. Lay the smoked salmon slices flat on a cutting board.

2. Disperse 1 tbsp. of cream cheese uniformly onto each salmon slice.
3. Sprinkle chopped chives over the cream cheese.
4. Roll up each slice firmly.
5. Cut every roll-up into smaller fragments using a sharp knife.
6. Serve chilled.

Per serving: Calories: 160kcal; Fat: 10g; Carbs: 2g; Protein: 14g; Sugar: 1g; Sodium: 450mg; Potassium: 220mg

57. Eggplant Lasagna Roll-Ups

Preparation time: 20 minutes

Cooking time: 40 minutes

Servings: 4

Ingredients:

- 2 big eggplants, finely cut lengthwise
- 1 cup ricotta cheese
- 1 cup marinara sauce
- 1 cup shredded mozzarella cheese
- 1/4 cup grated Parmesan cheese
- 2 tbsps. chopped fresh basil
- Salt and pepper as required

Directions:

1. Warm up oven to 375 deg.F.
2. Place eggplant slices on your baking sheet lined using parchment paper.
3. Sprinkle salt over the eggplant slices then let sit for 10 minutes to draw out some extra moisture.
4. Pat dry the eggplant slices using paper towels.
5. Put a fine layer of your marinara sauce over each eggplant slice.
6. Disperse ricotta cheese uniformly over each eggplant slice.
7. Roll up each eggplant slice then place seam side down in your baking dish.
8. Pour rest of the marinara sauce over the eggplant roll-ups.
9. Sprinkle your shredded mozzarella cheese and grated Parmesan cheese over the top.
10. Cover baking dish using foil then bake in to your warmed up oven for 30 minutes.
11. Take out foil then bake for extra 10 minutes, or 'til cheese is melted and bubbly.
12. Garnish using chopped fresh basil prior to presenting.

Per serving: Calories: 250kcal; Fat: 15g; Carbs: 15g; Protein: 15g; Sugar: 8g; Sodium: 600mg; Potassium: 800mg

58. Steak with Garlic Butter Mushrooms

Preparation time: 10 minutes

Cooking time: 15 minutes

Servings: 2

Ingredients:

- 2 beef steaks (e.g., sirloin or ribeye), about 8 oz each
- 2 tbsps. butter
- 2 pieces garlic, crushed
- 8 oz mushrooms, cut
- Salt and pepper as required
- Chopped fresh parsley for garnish

Directions:

1. Flavour beef steaks generously using salt and pepper on both sides.
2. Warm a skillet in a med-high temp.
3. Include beef steaks to your skillet then cook to your desired doneness, 4-5 minutes on all sides for medium-rare.
4. Take out steaks from the skillet then let rest for a couple of minutes.
5. In the similar skillet, melt butter in a middling temp.
6. Include crushed garlic to your skillet then cook 'til fragrant.
7. Include cut mushrooms to your skillet then cook 'til softened and browned.
8. Flavour mushrooms using salt and pepper as required.
9. Serve steaks topped with garlic butter mushrooms.
10. Garnish using chopped fresh parsley prior to presenting.

Per serving: Calories: 400kcal; Fat: 25g; Carbs: 5g; Protein: 40g; Sugar: 3g; Sodium: 300mg; Potassium: 800mg

59. Lemon Herb Baked Cod

Preparation time: 10 minutes

Cooking time: 20 minutes

Servings: 2

Ingredients:

- 2 cod fillets
- 2 tbsps. olive oil
- 2 pieces garlic, crushed
- Zest and juice of 1 lemon
- 1 tbsp. chopped fresh parsley

- 1 tsp. dried oregano
- Salt and pepper as required

Directions:

1. Warm up oven to 375 deg.F.
2. Place cod fillets in your baking dish lined using parchment paper.
3. In your small bowl, whisk collectively olive oil, crushed garlic, lemon zest, lemon juice, chopped fresh parsley, dried oregano, salt, and pepper.
4. Pour the lemon herb mixture over the cod fillets, ensuring they are uniformly coated.
5. Bake in to your warmed up oven for 15-20 minutes, or 'til fish is cooked through and flakes simply with a fork.
6. Present warm.

Per serving: Calories: 300kcal; Fat: 15g; Carbs: 2g; Protein: 35g; Sugar: 1g; Sodium: 400mg; Potassium: 800mg

60. Spaghetti Squash with Meatballs

Preparation time: 15 minutes

Cooking time: 1 hour

Servings: 4

Ingredients:

- 1 spaghetti squash
- 1 lb. lean ground beef
- 1/4 cup grated Parmesan cheese
- 1/4 cup almond flour
- 1 egg
- 1 tsp. Italian seasoning
- 1 cup marinara sauce
- Salt and pepper as required
- Fresh basil leaves for garnish

Directions:

1. Warm up oven to 375 deg.F.
2. Cut your spaghetti squash in half lengthwise then scoop out the seeds.
3. Place spaghetti squash halves cut side down on your baking sheet lined using parchment paper.
4. Bake in to your warmed up oven for 45-60 minutes, or 'til squash is tender and simply pierced with a fork.
5. While squash is baking, prepare the meatballs. In your bowl, blend ground beef, grated Parmesan cheese, almond flour, egg, Italian seasoning, salt, and pepper. Mix 'til well combined.
6. Roll the meat mixture into small meatballs.

7. In your skillet, brown the meatballs in a middling temp. 'til cooked through.
8. Heat marinara sauce in a saucepan in a middling temp.
9. Once cooked, use a fork to scrape the flesh into strands.
10. Serve spaghetti squash topped with meatballs and marinara sauce.
11. Garnish using fresh basil leaves prior to presenting.

Per serving: Calories: 350kcal; Fat: 20g; Carbs: 15g; Protein: 30g; Sugar: 5g; Sodium: 600mg; Potassium: 900mg

61. Stuffed Portobello Mushrooms with Spinach and Cheese

Preparation time: 20 minutes

Cooking time: 25 minutes

Servings: 4

Ingredients:

- 4 big portobello mushrooms, stems taken out
- 2 cups fresh spinach, chopped
- 1/2 cup ricotta cheese
- 1/4 cup grated Parmesan cheese
- 2 pieces garlic, crushed
- 1 tbsp. olive oil
- Salt and pepper as required
- Chopped fresh parsley for garnish

Directions:

1. Warm up oven to 375 deg.F.
2. Place portobello mushrooms on your baking sheet lined using parchment paper.
3. In your skillet, warm olive oil in a middling temp.
4. Include crushed garlic to your skillet then cook 'til fragrant.
5. Include chopped fresh spinach to your skillet then cook 'til wilted.
6. In your bowl, blend cooked spinach, ricotta cheese, grated Parmesan cheese, salt, and pepper.
7. Spoon the spinach mixture into the hollowed-out portobello mushrooms.
8. Bake in to your warmed up oven for 20-25 minutes, or 'til mushrooms are tender and filling is heated through.
9. Garnish using chopped fresh parsley prior to presenting.

Per serving: Calories: 150kcal; Fat: 8g; Carbs: 10g; Protein: 10g; Sugar: 3g; Sodium: 400mg; Potassium: 800mg

62. Chicken and Vegetable Stir-Fry

Preparation time: 15 minutes

Cooking time: 15 minutes

Servings: 2

Ingredients:

- 2 boneless, skinless chicken breasts, finely cut
- 1 bell pepper, finely cut
- 1 cup broccoli florets
- 1 carrot, finely cut
- 2 pieces garlic, crushed
- 2 tbsps. soy sauce
- 1 tbsp. oyster sauce
- 1 tbsp. olive oil
- Sesame seeds for garnish

Directions:

1. In your bowl, marinate finely cut chicken breasts with soy sauce and oyster sauce for 10 minutes.
2. Warm olive oil in your big skillet or wok at high temp.
3. Include crushed garlic to your skillet then cook 'til fragrant.
4. Include marinated chicken to your skillet then stir-fry 'til browned then cooked through.
5. Include cut bell pepper, broccoli florets, and finely cut carrot to your skillet.
6. Stir-fry vegetables with the chicken for 2-3 minutes, 'til tender-crisp.
7. Flavour using additional soy sauce or salt as required, if wanted.
8. Present warm, garnished with sesame seeds.

Per serving: Calories: 300kcal; Fat: 10g; Carbs: 15g; Protein: 30g; Sugar: 6g; Sodium: 900mg; Potassium: 800mg

63. Keto Chicken Parmesan

Preparation time: 15 minutes

Cooking time: 25 minutes

Servings: 2

Ingredients:

- 2 boneless, skinless chicken breasts
- 1/2 cup almond flour
- 1/4 cup grated Parmesan cheese
- 1 tsp. Italian seasoning
- 1 egg, beaten

- 1 cup marinara sauce
- 1/2 cup shredded mozzarella cheese
- 2 tbsps. chopped fresh basil
- Salt and pepper as required

Directions:

1. Warm up oven to 400 deg.F.
2. Flavour chicken breasts using salt and pepper on both sides.
3. In your shallow dish, blend almond flour, grated Parmesan cheese, and Italian seasoning.
4. Dip each chicken breast in your beaten egg, then coat with almond flour mixture.
5. Place coated chicken breasts in your baking dish lined using parchment paper.
6. Bake in to your warmed up oven for 20 minutes.
7. Take out chicken from the oven and spoon marinara sauce over each chicken breast.
8. Top with shredded mozzarella cheese.
9. Return to the oven then bake for extra 5 minutes, or 'til cheese is melted and bubbly.
10. Garnish using chopped fresh basil prior to presenting.

Per serving: Calories: 350kcal; Fat: 20g; Carbs: 10g; Protein: 30g; Sugar: 5g; Sodium: 800mg; Potassium: 800mg

64. Taco Stuffed Avocados

Preparation time: 15 minutes

Cooking time: 15 minutes

Servings: 4

Ingredients:

- 2 ripe avocados, divided and pitted
- 1 lb. ground beef
- 1 packet taco seasoning
- 1/2 cup diced tomatoes
- 1/4 cup diced red onion
- 1/4 cup shredded cheddar cheese
- 1/4 cup chopped fresh cilantro
- Lime wedges for presenting

Directions:

1. Warm up oven to 375 deg.F.
2. Scoop out a portion of avocado flesh from each avocado half to create a huge cavity.
3. In your skillet, cook ground beef in a middling temp. 'til browned then cooked through.
4. Drain extra fat from the skillet then stir in taco seasoning using the package guidelines.
5. Fill each avocado half with taco meat.

6. Top with diced tomatoes, diced red onion, shredded cheddar cheese, and chopped fresh cilantro.
7. Place stuffed avocado halves on your baking sheet lined using parchment paper.
8. Bake in to your warmed up oven for 10-12 minutes, or 'til your cheese is melted and bubbly.
9. Present warm with lime wedges.

Per serving: Calories: 350kcal; Fat: 25g; Carbs: 10g; Protein: 25g; Sugar: 3g; Sodium: 600mg; Potassium: 800mg

65. Greek Lemon Chicken Skewers

Preparation time: 15 minutes

Cooking time: 15 minutes

Servings: 4

Ingredients:

- 1 lb. boneless, skinless chicken breasts, chunks
- 1/4 cup olive oil
- Juice of 1 lemon
- Zest of 1 lemon
- 2 pieces garlic, crushed
- 1 tsp. dried oregano
- 1/2 tsp. dried thyme
- Salt and pepper as required
- Tzatziki sauce for presenting

Directions:

1. In your bowl, whisk collectively olive oil, lemon juice, lemon zest, crushed garlic, dried oregano, dried thyme, salt, and pepper.
2. Include chicken chunks to the bowl then toss to coat in the marinade.
3. Cover then put in the fridge chicken for almost 30 minutes, or up to 4 hours.
4. Warm up the grill pan to med-high temp.
5. Thread marinated chicken chunks onto skewers.
6. Grill your chicken skewers for 10-12 minutes, turning occasionally, 'til cooked through and mildly charred.
7. Present warm with tzatziki sauce for soaking.

Per serving: Calories: 250kcal; Fat: 15g; Carbs: 2g; Protein: 25g; Sugar: 1g; Sodium: 300mg; Potassium: 600mg

High Carb Dinner

66. Teriyaki Tofu Stir-Fry with Brown Rice

Preparation time: 15 minutes

Cooking time: 20 minutes

Servings: 4

Ingredients:

- 1 block firm tofu, pressed and cubed
- 2 cups mixed vegetables (e.g., broccoli, bell peppers, carrots)
- 1/4 cup teriyaki sauce
- 2 tbsps. soy sauce
- 1 tbsp. sesame oil
- 2 pieces garlic, crushed
- 1 tbsp. cornstarch
- Cooked brown rice, for presenting
- Sesame seeds and cut green onions (garnish)

Directions:

1. In your bowl, whisk collectively teriyaki sauce, soy sauce, sesame oil, crushed garlic, and cornstarch.
2. Warm a big skillet or wok in a med-high temp.
3. Include cubed tofu to your skillet then cook 'til browned and crispy on all sides.
4. Take out tofu from the skillet then put away.
5. In the similar skillet, include mixed vegetables then stir-fry 'til tender-crisp.
6. Return tofu to your skillet and pour the teriyaki sauce mixture over the tofu and vegetables.
7. Stir-fry for extra 2-3 minutes, 'til the sauce thickens and coats everything uniformly.
8. Present warm over cooked brown rice.
9. Garnish using sesame seeds and cut green onions.

Per serving: Calories: 300kcal; Fat: 12g; Carbs: 35g; Protein: 15g; Sugar: 8g; Sodium: 800mg; Potassium: 600mg

67. Vegetarian Chili with Whole Grain Bread

Preparation time: 15 minutes

Cooking time: 30 minutes

Servings: 6

Ingredients:

- 1 tbsp. olive oil
- 1 onion, diced

- 2 pieces garlic, crushed
- 1 bell pepper, diced
- 1 zucchini, diced
- 1 cup corn kernels (fresh or frozen)
- 15 oz black beans
- 15 oz kidney beans
- 15 oz diced tomatoes
- 2 cups vegetable broth
- 2 tbsps. chili powder
- 1 tsp. cumin
- Salt and pepper as required
- Chopped fresh cilantro for garnish
- Whole grain bread, for presenting

Directions:

1. Warm olive oil in your big pot in a middling temp.
2. Place diced onion and crushed garlic to the pot then cook 'til softened.
3. Stir in diced bell pepper and zucchini, then cook for an extra 5 minutes.
4. Include corn kernels, black beans, kidney beans, diced tomatoes, vegetable broth, chili powder, cumin, salt, and pepper to the pot.
5. Bring the chili to a simmer then let it cook for 20-25 minutes, mixing irregularly.
6. Adjust seasoning using more salt and pepper if wanted.
7. Present warm, garnished with chopped fresh cilantro.
8. Enjoy with slices of whole grain bread.

Per serving: Calories: 250kcal; Fat: 4g; Carbs: 45g; Protein: 12g; Sugar: 8g; Sodium: 700mg; Potassium: 900mg

68. Whole Wheat Pasta with Marinara Sauce

Preparation time: 10 minutes

Cooking time: 10 minutes

Servings: 4

Ingredients:

- 8 oz whole wheat pasta
- 2 cups marinara sauce
- 1 tbsp. olive oil
- 2 pieces garlic, crushed
- Salt and pepper as required
- Grated Parmesan cheese for garnish

- Chopped fresh basil for garnish

Directions:

1. Cook whole wheat pasta using the package guidelines 'til al dente. Drain then put away.
2. In your big skillet, warm olive oil in a middling temp.
3. Include crushed garlic to your skillet then cook 'til fragrant.
4. Pour marinara sauce into your skillet and heat 'til warmed through.
5. Include cooked pasta to your skillet then toss to coat uniformly with the sauce.
6. Flavour using salt and pepper as required.
7. Present warm, garnished using grated Parmesan cheese and chopped fresh basil.

Per serving: Calories: 300kcal; Fat: 5g; Carbs: 55g; Protein: 10g; Sugar: 8g; Sodium: 600mg; Potassium: 400mg

69. Chickpea Curry with Basmati Rice

Preparation time: 10 minutes

Cooking time: 25 minutes

Servings: 4

Ingredients:

- 1 cup basmati rice
- 15 oz chickpeas
- 1 onion, diced
- 2 pieces garlic, crushed
- 1 bell pepper, diced
- 1 zucchini, diced
- 15 oz diced tomatoes
- 13.5 oz coconut milk
- 2 tbsps. curry powder
- 1 tsp. ground turmeric
- Salt and pepper as required
- Chopped fresh cilantro for garnish

Directions:

1. Cook basmati rice using the package guidelines.
2. In your big skillet, warm olive oil in a middling temp.
3. Place diced onion and crushed garlic to your skillet then cook 'til softened.
4. Stir in diced bell pepper and zucchini, then cook for an extra 5 minutes.
5. Include chickpeas, diced tomatoes, coconut milk, curry powder, ground turmeric, salt, and pepper to your skillet.

6. Simmer curry for 10-15 minutes, mixing irregularly, 'til vegetables are tender and flavors are combined.
7. Adjust seasoning using more salt and pepper if wanted.
8. Present warm over cooked basmati rice.
9. Garnish using chopped fresh cilantro.

Per serving: Calories: 350kcal; Fat: 10g; Carbs: 55g; Protein: 12g; Sugar: 8g; Sodium: 700mg; Potassium: 800mg

70. Quinoa Stuffed Bell Peppers

Preparation time: 15 minutes
Cooking time: 40 minutes
Servings: 4
Ingredients:

- 4 bell peppers, tops taken out and seeds taken out
- 1 cup quinoa, cooked
- 15 oz black beans
- 1 cup corn kernels (fresh or frozen)
- 1 cup diced tomatoes
- 1/2 cup shredded cheddar cheese
- 1 tsp. chili powder
- 1/2 tsp. cumin
- Salt and pepper as required
- Chopped fresh cilantro for garnish

Directions:
1. Warm up oven to 375 deg.F.
2. In your big bowl, blend cooked quinoa, black beans, corn kernels, diced tomatoes, shredded cheddar cheese, chili powder, cumin, salt, and pepper.
3. Stuff each bell pepper using the quinoa mixture.
4. Place stuffed bell peppers in your baking dish.
5. Cover the baking dish using foil then bake in to your warmed up oven for 30 minutes.
6. Take out foil then bake for extra 10 minutes, or 'til peppers are tender and filling is heated through.
7. Present warm, garnished with chopped fresh cilantro.

Per serving: Calories: 300kcal; Fat: 5g; Carbs: 50g; Protein: 12g; Sugar: 8g; Sodium: 600mg; Potassium: 800mg

71. Veggie Stir-Fry with Rice Noodles

Preparation time: 15 minutes

Cooking time: 15 minutes

Servings: 4

Ingredients:

- 8 oz rice noodles
- 2 tbsps. sesame oil
- 2 pieces garlic, crushed
- 1 onion, finely cut
- 2 carrots, julienned
- 1 bell pepper, finely cut
- 1 cup snow peas, trimmed
- 1/4 cup soy sauce
- 2 tbsps. rice vinegar
- 1 tbsp. honey
- 1 tsp. grated ginger
- Salt and pepper as required
- Sesame seeds for garnish

Directions:

1. Cook rice noodles using the package guidelines. Drain then put away.
2. In your big skillet or wok, heat sesame oil in a med-high temp.
3. Include crushed garlic and finely cut onion to your skillet then cook 'til softened.
4. Stir in julienned carrots, finely cut bell pepper, and trimmed snow peas.
5. Cook vegetables for 5-7 minutes, 'til tender-crisp.
6. In your small bowl, whisk collectively soy sauce, rice vinegar, honey, and grated ginger.
7. Place the sauce over the cooked vegetables in the skillet.
8. Include cooked rice noodles to your skillet then toss everything together 'til uniformly coated with the sauce.
9. Flavour using salt and pepper as required.
10. Present warm, garnished with sesame seeds.

Per serving: Calories: 350kcal; Fat: 5g; Carbs: 65g; Protein: 8g; Sugar: 8g; Sodium: 800mg; Potassium: 600mg

72. Butternut Squash Risotto

Preparation time: 10 minutes

Cooking time: 30 minutes

Servings: 4

Ingredients:

- 1 tbsp. olive oil
- 1 small onion, diced
- 2 pieces garlic, crushed
- 1 cup Arborio rice
- 3 cups vegetable broth, warmed
- 2 cups diced butternut squash
- 1/4 cup grated Parmesan cheese
- Salt and pepper as required
- Chopped fresh sage for garnish

Directions:

1. Warm olive oil in your big skillet or pot in a middling temp.
2. Include diced onion to your skillet then cook 'til softened.
3. Stir in crushed garlic and Arborio rice, then cook for an extra 2 minutes.
4. Include diced butternut squash to your skillet.
5. Gradually include warmed vegetable broth to your skillet, ½ cup at a time, mixing regularly then allowing the liquid to be immersed before placing more.
6. Continue cooking then mixing 'til the rice is creamy and tender, and butternut squash is cooked through, about 20-25 minutes.
7. Stir in grated Parmesan cheese then flavour using salt and pepper as required.
8. Present warm, garnished with chopped fresh sage.

Per serving: Calories: 300kcal; Fat: 5g; Carbs: 55g; Protein: 8g; Sugar: 8g; Sodium: 700mg; Potassium: 600mg

73. Whole Grain Pizza with Vegetables

Preparation time: 15 minutes

Cooking time: 20 minutes

Servings: 4

Ingredients:

- 1 pre-made whole grain pizza dough
- 1/2 cup marinara sauce
- 1 cup shredded mozzarella cheese
- 1 bell pepper, finely cut
- 1/2 red onion, finely cut
- 1 cup cut mushrooms
- 1 cup spinach leaves
- 1 tbsp. olive oil
- Salt and pepper as required

- Crushed red pepper flakes for garnish

Directions:

1. Warm up oven to 425 deg.F.
2. Roll out whole grain pizza dough on your baking sheet lined using parchment paper.
3. Disperse marinara sauce uniformly over your pizza dough.
4. Sprinkle shredded mozzarella cheese over the sauce.
5. Organize finely cut bell pepper, red onion, cut mushrooms, and spinach leaves on top of the cheese.
6. Drizzle olive oil over your vegetables then flavour using salt and pepper as required.
7. Bake in to your warmed up oven for 15-20 minutes, or 'til crust is golden brown and cheese is melted and bubbly.
8. Sprinkle crushed red pepper flakes over your pizza prior to presenting.

Per serving: Calories: 350kcal; Fat: 10g; Carbs: 55g; Protein: 15g; Sugar: 8g; Sodium: 700mg; Potassium: 600mg

74. *Black Bean Enchiladas with Brown Rice*

Preparation time: 20 minutes

Cooking time: 25 minutes

Servings: 4

Ingredients:

- 15 oz black beans
- 1 cup corn kernels (fresh or frozen)
- 1 bell pepper, diced
- 1/2 red onion, diced
- 2 pieces garlic, crushed
- 1 tsp. chili powder
- 1/2 tsp. cumin
- Salt and pepper as required
- 8 whole wheat tortillas
- 1 cup enchilada sauce
- 1 cup shredded cheddar cheese
- Chopped fresh cilantro for garnish

Directions:

1. Warm up oven to 375 deg.F.
2. In your big skillet, warm olive oil in a middling temp.
3. Include diced bell pepper and diced red onion to your skillet then cook 'til softened.
4. Stir in crushed garlic, chili powder, and cumin, then cook 'til fragrant.

5. Include black beans and corn kernels to your skillet, then flavour using salt and pepper as required. Cook for 5 minutes.

6. Warm whole wheat tortillas using the package guidelines.

7. Put a spoonful of enchilada sauce on each tortilla.

8. Spoon black bean mixture onto each tortilla and roll up firmly.

9. Place rolled enchiladas seam-side down in a baking dish.

10. Place rest of the enchilada sauce over the top of the enchiladas.

11. Sprinkle shredded cheddar cheese over the sauce.

12. Bake in to your warmed up oven for 20-25 minutes, or 'til your cheese is melted and bubbly.

13. Present warm, garnished with chopped fresh cilantro.

Per serving: Calories: 400kcal; Fat: 10g; Carbs: 60g; Protein: 15g; Sugar: 8g; Sodium: 800mg; Potassium: 600mg

75. Spinach and Feta Stuffed Peppers with Couscous

Preparation time: 15 minutes

Cooking time: 30 minutes

Servings: 4

Ingredients:

- 4 big bell peppers, tops taken out and seeds taken out
- 1 cup couscous, cooked
- 2 cups fresh spinach leaves
- 1/2 cup crumbled feta cheese
- 1/4 cup chopped sun-dried tomatoes
- 2 pieces garlic, crushed
- 1 tbsp. olive oil
- Salt and pepper as required
- Chopped fresh parsley for garnish

Directions:

1. Warm up oven to 375 deg.F.

2. In your skillet, warm olive oil in a middling temp.

3. Include crushed garlic to your skillet then cook 'til fragrant.

4. Include fresh spinach leaves to your skillet then cook 'til wilted.

5. In your bowl, blend cooked couscous, wilted spinach, crumbled feta cheese, chopped sun-dried tomatoes, salt, and pepper.

6. Stuff each bell pepper using the couscous mixture.

7. Place stuffed peppers in a baking dish.

8. Cover the baking dish using foil then bake in to your warmed up oven for 25 minutes.

9. Take out foil then bake for extra 5 minutes, or 'til peppers are tender.
10. Present warm, garnished with chopped fresh parsley.

Per serving: Calories: 350kcal; Fat: 10g; Carbs: 50g; Protein: 12g; Sugar: 8g; Sodium: 700mg; Potassium: 800mg

76. Lentil and Vegetable Soup with Whole Grain Bread

Preparation time: 15 minutes

Cooking time: 30 minutes

Servings: 6

Ingredients:

- 1 cup dry green lentils
- 1 onion, diced
- 2 carrots, diced
- 2 celery stalks, diced
- 2 pieces garlic, crushed
- 15 oz diced tomatoes
- 6 cups vegetable broth
- 1 tsp. dried thyme
- 1 tsp. dried oregano
- Salt and pepper as required
- Chopped fresh parsley for garnish
- Cuts of whole grain bread, for presenting

Directions:

1. Rinse dry green lentils under cold water then drain.
2. In your big pot, warm olive oil in a middling temp.
3. Include diced onion, diced carrots, diced celery, and crushed garlic to the pot. Cook 'til softened.
4. Stir in diced tomatoes, vegetable broth, dried thyme, dried oregano, salt, pepper, then drained lentils.
5. Boil the soup, then decrease temp. then simmer for 25-30 minutes, or 'til lentils and vegetables are tender.
6. Adjust seasoning using more salt and pepper if wanted.
7. Present warm, garnished with chopped fresh parsley.
8. Enjoy with slices of whole grain bread.

Per serving: Calories: 300kcal; Fat: 5g; Carbs: 50g; Protein: 15g; Sugar: 8g; Sodium: 800mg; Potassium: 800mg

77. Sweet Potato and Chickpea Buddha Bowl

Preparation time: 15 minutes

Cooking time: 25 minutes

Servings: 4

Ingredients:

- 2 big sweet potatoes, skinned and cubed
- 15 oz chickpeas
- 2 cups broccoli florets
- 2 tbsps. olive oil
- 1 tsp. smoked paprika
- 1/2 tsp. cumin
- Salt and pepper as required
- 2 cups cooked quinoa
- 1 avocado, cut
- 1/4 cup hummus
- Chopped fresh parsley for garnish

Directions:

1. Warm up oven to 400 deg.F.
2. In your bowl, toss cubed sweet potatoes, drained chickpeas, and broccoli florets with olive oil, smoked paprika, cumin, salt, and pepper.
3. Place the seasoned vegetables in a single layer on your baking sheet lined using parchment paper.
4. Roast in to your warmed up oven for 20-25 minutes, or 'til vegetables are tender and mildly caramelized.
5. Divide cooked quinoa among serving bowls.
6. Top with roasted sweet potatoes, chickpeas, and broccoli.
7. Include cut avocado and a dollop of hummus to each bowl.
8. Garnish using chopped fresh parsley.
9. Present warm or at room temp.

Per serving: Calories: 400kcal; Fat: 15g; Carbs: 60g; Protein: 15g; Sugar: 8g; Sodium: 600mg; Potassium: 800mg

78. Vegetable Paella

Preparation time: 15 minutes

Cooking time: 35 minutes

Servings: 4

Ingredients:

- 1 tbsp. olive oil
- 1 onion, diced
- 2 pieces garlic, crushed
- 1 bell pepper, diced
- 1 zucchini, diced
- 1 cup cherry tomatoes, divided
- 1 cup frozen peas
- 1 1/2 cups Arborio rice
- 3 cups vegetable broth
- 1 tsp. smoked paprika
- 1/2 tsp. saffron threads (optional)
- Salt and pepper as required
- Chopped fresh parsley for garnish

Directions:

1. In your big skillet or paella pan, warm olive oil in a middling temp.
2. Include diced onion to your skillet then cook 'til softened.
3. Stir in crushed garlic, diced bell pepper, and diced zucchini, then cook for an extra 5 minutes.
4. Include divided cherry tomatoes and frozen peas to your skillet, then cook for 2-3 minutes.
5. Stir in Arborio rice, smoked paprika, saffron threads (if using), salt, and pepper.
6. Pour vegetable broth in to your skillet then stir to blend.
7. Simmer the mixture, then decrease temp. to low and cover.
8. Cook for 20-25 minutes, or 'til rice is tender and liquid is immersed, mixing irregularly.
9. Adjust seasoning using more salt and pepper if wanted.
10. Present warm, garnished with chopped fresh parsley.

Per serving: Calories: 350kcal; Fat: 5g; Carbs: 65g; Protein: 8g; Sugar: 8g; Sodium: 800mg; Potassium: 600mg

79. Corn and Black Bean Quesadillas

Preparation time: 10 minutes

Cooking time: 15 minutes

Servings: 4

Ingredients:

- 8 whole wheat tortillas
- 1 cup corn kernels (fresh or frozen)
- 15 oz black beans
- 1 bell pepper, diced
- 1/2 red onion, diced

- 1 tsp. chili powder
- 1/2 tsp. cumin
- Salt and pepper as required
- 1 cup shredded cheddar cheese
- Salsa, guacamole, and sour cream for presenting

Directions:
1. In your skillet, warm olive oil in a middling temp.
2. Include diced bell pepper and diced red onion to your skillet then cook 'til softened.
3. Stir in corn kernels, drained black beans, chili powder, cumin, salt, and pepper. Cook for 5 minutes.
4. Warm whole wheat tortillas using the package guidelines.
5. Disperse a spoonful of black bean mixture on one half of each tortilla.
6. Sprinkle shredded cheddar cheese over the black bean mixture.
7. Fold the other half of the tortilla over the filling to form a half-moon shape.
8. Repeat with rest of the tortillas and filling.
9. In your clean skillet, cook quesadillas in a middling temp. for 2-3 minutes on all sides, or 'til golden brown and crispy.
10. Cut quesadillas into wedges then serve hot with salsa, guacamole, and sour cream.

Per serving: Calories: 400kcal; Fat: 15g; Carbs: 50g; Protein: 15g; Sugar: 8g; Sodium: 700mg; Potassium: 600mg

80. Barley Salad with Roasted Vegetables

Preparation time: 15 minutes

Cooking time: 30 minutes

Servings: 4

Ingredients:

- 1 cup pearl barley
- 2 cups vegetable broth
- 1 sweet potato, skinned and cubed
- 1 red bell pepper, diced
- 1 zucchini, diced
- 1 cup cherry tomatoes, divided
- 1/4 cup chopped fresh parsley
- 2 tbsps. olive oil
- 1 tbsp. balsamic vinegar
- Salt and pepper as required
- Crumbled feta cheese for garnish

Directions:

1. Warm up oven to 400 deg.F.
2. Rinse pearl barley under cold water then drain.
3. In your saucepan, bring vegetable broth to a boil.
4. Include pearl barley to the boiling broth, decrease temp. to low, cover, then simmer for 25-30 minutes, or 'til barley is tender and liquid is immersed.
5. In the meantime, spread cubed sweet potato, diced red bell pepper, diced zucchini, and divided cherry tomatoes on your baking sheet lined using parchment paper.
6. Drizzle your olive oil and balsamic vinegar over the vegetables, then flavour using salt and pepper as required.
7. Toss to coat uniformly, then roast in to your warmed up oven for 20-25 minutes, or 'til vegetables are tender and caramelized.
8. In your big bowl, blend cooked pearl barley, roasted vegetables, and chopped fresh parsley.
9. Adjust seasoning using more salt and pepper if wanted.
10. Present warm or at room temp., garnished using crumbled feta cheese.

Per serving: Calories: 350kcal; Fat: 10g; Carbs: 60g; Protein: 10g; Sugar: 8g; Sodium: 700mg; Potassium: 600mg

Snacks and Smoothies Recipes

Low Carb Snacks

81. Caprese Skewers

Preparation time: 10 minutes

Servings: 4

Ingredients:

- 8 cherry tomatoes
- 8 fresh mozzarella balls (bocconcini)
- 8 fresh basil leaves
- Balsamic glaze, for drizzling
- Salt and pepper as required

Directions:

1. Thread a cherry tomato, a mozzarella ball, and a basil leaf onto a small skewer.
2. Repeat with the rest of the components 'til you have 8 skewers.
3. Organize the skewers on a serving platter.
4. Drizzle using balsamic glaze.
5. Flavour using salt and pepper as required.
6. Present instantly.

Per serving: Calories: 90kcal; Fat: 6g; Carbs: 3g; Protein: 6g; Sugar: 2g; Sodium: 150mg; Potassium: 120mg

82. Stuffed Mini Bell Peppers

Preparation time: 15 minutes

Cooking time: 15 minutes

Servings: 4

Ingredients:

- 12 mini bell peppers, divided and seeds taken out
- 1 cup cream cheese, softened
- 1/2 cup shredded cheddar cheese
- 2 green onions, finely cut
- 1 tsp. garlic powder
- Salt and pepper as required

Directions:

1. Warm up oven to 375 deg.F.

2. In mixing bowl, blend softened cream cheese, shredded cheddar cheese, cut green onions, garlic powder, salt, and pepper.
3. Fill each divided mini bell pepper with the cream cheese mixture.
4. Place stuffed mini bell peppers on your baking sheet lined using parchment paper.
5. Bake in to your warmed up oven for 12-15 minutes, or 'til peppers are tender and filling is heated through.
6. Take out from the oven then let cool mildly prior to presenting.

Per serving: Calories: 150kcal; Fat: 12g; Carbs: 6g; Protein: 5g; Sugar: 3g; Sodium: 200mg; Potassium: 300mg

83. Cauliflower Hummus

Preparation time: 10 minutes

Cooking time: 25 minutes

Servings: 4

Ingredients:

- 1 small head cauliflower, cut into florets
- 2 pieces garlic, crushed
- 2 tbsps. tahini
- 2 tbsps. lemon juice
- 2 tbsps. olive oil
- 1/2 tsp. ground cumin
- Salt and pepper as required
- Optional: chopped fresh parsley for garnish

Directions:

1. Warm up oven to 400 deg.F.
2. Place cauliflower florets on your baking sheet lined using parchment paper.
3. Drizzle using olive oil then flavour using salt and pepper as required.
4. Roast in to your warmed up oven for 20-25 minutes, or 'til cauliflower is tender and golden brown.
5. Transfer roasted cauliflower to a blending container.
6. Include crushed garlic, tahini, lemon juice, and ground cumin to the blending container.
7. Pulse 'til smooth and creamy, scraping down the sides as needed.
8. Adjust seasoning using more salt and pepper if wanted.
9. Transfer cauliflower hummus to a serving bowl.
10. Garnish using chopped fresh parsley if desired.

Per serving: Calories: 90kcal; Fat: 7g; Carbs: 5g; Protein: 3g; Sugar: 2g; Sodium: 150mg; Potassium: 280mg

84. Eggplant Chips

Preparation time: 10 minutes

Cooking time: 20 minutes

Servings: 4

Ingredients:

- 1 big eggplant, finely cut
- 2 tbsps. olive oil
- 1 tsp. Italian seasoning
- Salt and pepper as required

Directions:

1. Warm up oven to 375 deg.F.
2. Place eggplant slices on your baking sheet lined using parchment paper.
3. Drizzle olive oil over the eggplant slices.
4. Sprinkle your Italian seasoning, salt, and pepper over the slices.
5. Bake in to your warmed up oven for 15-20 minutes, or 'til eggplant chips are golden brown and crispy.
6. Take out from the oven then let cool mildly prior to presenting.

Per serving: Calories: 60kcal; Fat: 5g; Carbs: 4g; Protein: 1g; Sugar: 2g; Sodium: 150mg; Potassium: 200mg

85. Cottage Cheese and Tomato Cuts

Preparation time: 5 minutes

Servings: 2

Ingredients:

- 1 cup cottage cheese
- 1 big tomato, cut
- Salt and pepper as required
- Optional: fresh basil leaves for garnish

Directions:

1. Place cottage cheese in a serving bowl.
2. Organize tomato slices on a plate.
3. Sprinkle tomato slices using salt and pepper as required.
4. Serve cottage cheese alongside tomato slices.
5. Garnish using fresh basil leaves if desired.

Per serving: Calories: 120kcal; Fat: 5g; Carbs: 7g; Protein: 12g; Sugar: 5g; Sodium: 300mg; Potassium: 400mg

86. Cucumber and Cream Cheese Bites

Preparation time: 10 minutes

Servings: 4

Ingredients:

- 1 cucumber, cut into rounds
- 1/2 cup cream cheese, softened
- 2 tbsps. chopped fresh dill
- Salt and pepper as required

Directions:

1. Disperse a fine layer of your softened cream cheese on each cucumber round.
2. Sprinkle chopped fresh dill over the cream cheese.
3. Flavour using salt and pepper as required.
4. Present instantly.

Per serving: Calories: 60kcal; Fat: 5g; Carbs: 3g; Protein: 2g; Sugar: 2g; Sodium: 150mg; Potassium: 200mg

87. Stuffed Celery Sticks

Preparation time: 10 minutes

Servings: 4

Ingredients:

- 4 celery stalks, cut into sticks
- 1/2 cup cream cheese, softened
- 2 tbsps. chopped fresh chives
- Salt and pepper as required

Directions:

1. In your bowl, mix softened cream cheese with chopped fresh chives.
2. Disperse the cream cheese mixture onto celery sticks.
3. Flavour using salt and pepper as required.
4. Present instantly.

Per serving: Calories: 70kcal; Fat: 6g; Carbs: 2g; Protein: 2g; Sugar: 1g; Sodium: 100mg; Potassium: 200mg

High Carb Snacks

88. *Hummus and Veggie Wrap*

Preparation time: 10 minutes

Servings: 1

Ingredients:

- 1 big whole grain wrap
- 2 tbsps. hummus
- 1/4 cup shredded carrots
- 1/4 cup cut cucumber
- 1/4 cup cut bell peppers
- 1/4 cup baby spinach leaves

Directions:

1. Lay the whole grain wrap on a clean surface.
2. Disperse hummus uniformly over the entire surface of the wrap.
3. Layer shredded carrots, cut cucumber, cut bell peppers, then baby spinach leaves on top of the hummus.
4. Roll the wrap firmly, tucking in the sides as you go.
5. Cut your wrap in half or into bite-sized pieces.
6. Present instantly.

Per serving: Calories: 250kcal; Fat: 7g; Carbs: 40g; Protein: 9g; Fiber: 7g; Sugar: 5g; Sodium: 400mg; Potassium: 600mg

89. *Fruit and Yogurt Parfait*

Preparation time: 5 minutes

Servings: 1

Ingredients:

- 1/2 cup Greek yogurt
- 1/4 cup granola
- 1/4 cup mixed fresh berries (e.g., strawberries, blueberries, raspberries)
- 1 tbsp. honey (optional)

Directions:

1. In your serving glass or bowl, layer Greek yogurt, granola, and mixed fresh berries.
2. Repeat the layers 'til the glass or bowl is filled.
3. Drizzle honey over the top if desired.
4. Present instantly.

Per serving: Calories: 300kcal; Fat: 6g; Carbs: 50g; Protein: 15g; Fiber: 5g; Sugar: 25g; Sodium: 100mg; Potassium: 300mg

90. Baked Sweet Potato Fries

Preparation time: 10 minutes

Cooking time: 25 minutes

Servings: 2

Ingredients:

- 2 medium sweet potatoes, cut into fries
- 1 tbsp. olive oil
- 1/2 tsp. paprika
- 1/2 tsp. garlic powder
- Salt and pepper as required

Directions:

1. Warm up oven to 425 deg.F.
2. In your big bowl, toss sweet potato fries with olive oil, paprika, garlic powder, salt, and pepper 'til uniformly coated.
3. Disperse the fries in a single layer on your baking sheet lined using parchment paper.
4. Bake in to your warmed up oven for 20-25 minutes, flipping halfway through, 'til fries are golden brown and crispy.
5. Take out from the oven then let cool mildly prior to presenting.
6. Serve with your favorite dipping sauce.

Per serving: Calories: 200kcal; Fat: 7g; Carbs: 35g; Protein: 3g; Fiber: 5g; Sugar: 8g; Sodium: 200mg; Potassium: 500mg

91. Banana Nut Muffins

Preparation time: 15 minutes

Cooking time: 20 minutes

Servings: 12

Ingredients:

- 2 cups whole wheat flour
- 1 tsp. baking powder
- 1/2 tsp. baking soda
- 1/2 tsp. salt
- 1/2 cup unsalted butter, melted
- 1/2 cup honey
- 2 eggs

- 3 ripe bananas, mashed
- 1/2 cup chopped walnuts
- 1 tsp. vanilla extract

Directions:

1. Warm up oven to 350 deg.F. Line a muffin tin with paper liners.
2. In your big bowl, whisk collectively whole wheat flour, baking powder, baking soda, and salt.
3. In another bowl, mix melted butter, honey, eggs, mashed bananas, chopped walnuts, and vanilla extract 'til well combined.
4. Pour the wet components in to your dry components then stir 'til just combined.
5. Spoon the batter in to your prepared muffin tin, filling each cup about 2/3 full.
6. Bake in to your warmed up oven for 18-20 minutes, or 'til a toothpick immersed in to your center comes out clean.
7. Take out from the oven then let cool in your muffin tin for 5 minutes before placing to your wire rack to cool entirely.

Per serving: Calories: 200kcal; Fat: 8g; Carbs: 30g; Protein: 4g; Fiber: 3g; Sugar: 14g; Sodium: 150mg; Potassium: 200mg

92. Banana Bread

Preparation time: 15 minutes

Cooking time: 50 minutes

Servings: 10

Ingredients:

- 3 ripe bananas, mashed
- 1/3 cup melted butter
- 3/4 cup granulated sugar
- 1 egg, beaten
- 1 tsp. vanilla extract
- 1 tsp. baking soda
- 1/4 salt
- 1 1/2 cups all-purpose flour

Directions:

1. Warm up oven to 350 deg.F. Grease a 9x5-inch loaf pan.
2. In your mixing bowl, blend mashed bananas and melted butter.
3. Place granulated sugar, beaten egg, and vanilla extract. Mix well.
4. Sprinkle your baking soda and salt over the mixture then stir to incorporate.
5. Gradually include all-purpose flour to the mixture, mixing 'til just combined.
6. Pour batter into your prepared loaf pan.

7. Bake in to your warmed up oven for 50-60 minutes, or 'til a toothpick placed into the center comes out clean.
8. Let the banana bread to cool in the pan for 10 minutes before transferring to your wire rack to cool entirely.
9. Cut and serve.

Per serving: Calories: 230kcal; Fat: 7g; Carbs: 39g; Protein: 3g; Fiber: 2g; Sugar: 20g; Sodium: 200mg; Potassium: 200mg

93. *Whole Grain Toast with Jam*

Preparation time: 5 minutes

Servings: 2

Ingredients:

- 2 slices whole grain bread, toasted
- 2 tbsps. fruit jam or preserves (e.g., strawberry or raspberry)

Directions:

1. Toast the whole grain bread slices 'til golden brown.
2. Disperse fruit jam or preserves uniformly over each slice of toast.
3. Present instantly.

Per serving: Calories: 150kcal; Fat: 1g; Carbs: 32g; Protein: 4g; Fiber: 3g; Sugar: 16g; Sodium: 200mg; Potassium: 100mg

94. *Chocolate Banana Oat Bars*

Preparation time: 15 minutes

Cooking time: 25 minutes

Servings: 12

Ingredients:

- 2 ripe bananas, mashed
- 1/4 cup honey
- 1/4 cup unsweetened applesauce
- 1 tsp. vanilla extract
- 2 cups rolled oats
- 1/4 cup cocoa powder
- 1/4 cup chocolate chips (optional)

Directions:

1. Warm up oven to 350 deg.F. Grease an 8x8-inch baking dish.
2. In your mixing bowl, blend mashed bananas, honey, unsweetened applesauce, and vanilla extract.
3. Stir in rolled oats and cocoa powder 'til well combined.

4. If using, fold in chocolate chips.
5. Press the mixture uniformly in to your prepared baking dish.
6. Bake in to your warmed up oven for 20-25 minutes, or 'til the edges are golden brown.
7. Let the bars to cool in the baking dish before cutting into squares.
8. Store leftovers in a sealed container.

Per serving: Calories: 120kcal; Fat: 2g; Carbs: 25g; Protein: 3g; Fiber: 3g; Sugar: 10g; Sodium: 0mg; Potassium: 150mg

Low Carb Smoothies

95. Creamy Vanilla Almond Smoothie

Preparation time: 5 minutes

Servings: 1

Ingredients:

- 1/2 cup unsweetened almond milk
- 1/4 cup Greek yogurt
- 1/4 cup heavy cream
- 1/2 tsp. vanilla extract
- 1 tbsp. almond butter
- 1/2 tsp. cinnamon
- Ice cubes (optional)

Directions:

1. In your blender, blend almond milk, Greek yogurt, heavy cream, vanilla extract, almond butter, and cinnamon.
2. If desired, place ice cubes for a colder smoothie.
3. Blend 'til smooth and creamy.
4. Pour into a glass and serve immediately.

Per serving: Calories: 250kcal; Fat: 22g; Carbs: 6g; Protein: 8g; Fiber: 2g; Sugar: 2g; Sodium: 80mg; Potassium: 200mg

96. Coconut Lime Green Smoothie

Preparation time: 5 minutes

Servings: 1

Ingredients:

- 1/2 cup unsweetened coconut milk
- 1/2 avocado

- Juice of 1 lime
- Handful of spinach
- 1 tbsp. chia seeds
- Ice cubes (optional)

Directions:

1. In your blender, blend coconut milk, avocado, lime juice, spinach, and chia seeds.
2. If desired, place ice cubes for a colder smoothie.
3. Blend 'til smooth and creamy.
4. Pour into a glass and serve immediately.

Per serving: Calories: 250kcal; Fat: 21g; Carbs: 12g; Protein: 6g; Fiber: 9g; Sugar: 1g; Sodium: 20mg; Potassium: 480mg

97. Coffee Protein Shake

Preparation time: 5 minutes

Servings: 1

Ingredients:

- 1/2 cup brewed coffee, cooled
- 1/2 cup unsweetened almond milk
- 1 scoop chocolate protein powder
- 1 tbsp. almond butter
- Ice cubes (optional)

Directions:

1. In your blender, blend cooled brewed coffee, almond milk, chocolate protein powder, and almond butter.
2. If desired, place ice cubes for a colder shake.
3. Blend 'til smooth and creamy.
4. Pour into a glass and serve immediately.

Per serving: Calories: 200kcal; Fat: 9g; Carbs: 6g; Protein: 25g; Fiber: 2g; Sugar: 2g; Sodium: 200mg; Potassium: 300mg

High Carb Smoothies

98. Pineapple Coconut Smoothie Bowl

Preparation time: 5 minutes

Servings: 1

Ingredients:

- 1 cup frozen pineapple chunks
- 1/2 cup coconut milk
- 1/2 banana
- 1 tbsp. shredded coconut
- 1 tbsp. chia seeds
- Cutd banana, strawberries, and granola for topping (optional)

Directions:

1. In your blender, blend frozen pineapple chunks, coconut milk, half a banana, shredded coconut, and chia seeds.
2. Blend 'til smooth and creamy.
3. Pour the smoothie into a bowl.
4. Top with cut banana, strawberries, and granola if desired.
5. Present instantly with a spoon.

Per serving: Calories: 380kcal; Fat: 20g; Carbs: 50g; Protein: 5g; Fiber: 8g; Sugar: 32g; Sodium: 30mg; Potassium: 560mg

99. Peach Raspberry Smoothie

Preparation time: 5 minutes

Servings: 1

Ingredients:

- 1 ripe peach, pitted and cut
- 1/2 cup fresh or frozen raspberries
- 1/2 cup Greek yogurt
- 1/2 cup orange juice
- 1 tbsp. honey (optional)
- Ice cubes (optional)

Directions:

1. In your blender, blend ripe peach slices, raspberries, Greek yogurt, orange juice, and honey (if using).
2. If desired, place ice cubes for a colder smoothie.
3. Blend 'til smooth and creamy.

4. Pour into a glass and serve immediately.

Per serving: Calories: 280kcal; Fat: 2g; Carbs: 60g; Protein: 11g; Fiber: 8g; Sugar: 45g; Sodium: 35mg; Potassium: 650mg

100. *Mango Banana Smoothie Bowl*

Preparation time: 5 minutes

Servings: 1

Ingredients:

- 1 ripe banana
- 1/2 cup frozen mango chunks
- 1/2 cup Greek yogurt
- 1/2 cup orange juice
- Cutd banana, mango, and granola for topping (optional)

Directions:

1. In your blender, blend ripe banana, frozen mango chunks, Greek yogurt, and orange juice.
2. Blend 'til smooth and creamy.
3. Pour the smoothie into a bowl.
4. Top with cut banana, mango, and granola if desired.
5. Present instantly with a spoon.

Per serving: Calories: 280kcal; Fat: 1g; Carbs: 65g; Protein: 12g; Fiber: 6g; Sugar: 45g; Sodium: 60mg; Potassium: 850mg

30 Days Meal Plan

Day	Breakfast	Lunch	Snack	Dinner	Type of Exercise	Exercise Description	Carb Cycling
1	Bacon and Egg Muffins	Tuna Salad Stuffed Bell Peppers	Cottage Cheese and Tomato Cuts	Smoked Salmon Roll-Ups	Strength Training	Full-body strength training with comlb. exercises such as squats, deadlifts, bench press, and rows. Aim for 3 sets of 8-12 reps.	Low
2	Buckwheat Pancakes with Berries	Whole Wheat Pita Pizza	Fruit and Yogurt Parfait	Butternut Squash Risotto	HIIT Cardio	HIIT with exercises like sprints, burpees, and jumping jacks. Alternate between periods of high intensity and rest for 20-30 minutes.	High
3	Avocado Egg Salad	Chicken Caesar Lettuce Wraps	Stuffed Mini Bell Peppers	Stuffed Portobello Mushrooms with Spinach and Cheese	Yoga/Pilates	Focus on flexibility and core strength through yoga or Pilates routines. Include poses like downward dog, plank, warrior series, and bridges.	Low
4	Multigrain Waffles with Honey	Sweet Potato and Black Bean Quesadilla	Chocolate Banana Oat Bars	Spinach and Feta Stuffed Peppers with Couscous	Cardio	Moderate-intensity cardio exercise such as jogging, cycling, or swimming for 30-45 minutes. Maintain a steady pace to increase heart rate and burn calories.	High

5	Cauliflower Breakfast Hash	Keto Eggplant Parmesan	Stuffed Celery Sticks	Beef and Broccoli Stir-Fry	Circuit Training	Circuit training incorporating both strength and cardio exercises. Perform a series of bodyweight exercises like lunges, push-ups, jumping rope, and mountain climbers for 3 rounds with minimal rest.	Low
6	Whole Wheat Pancakes with Maple Syrup	Whole Grain Pasta Salad with Pesto	Banana Nut Muffins	Whole Wheat Pasta with Marinara Sauce	Active Rest	Engage in light physical activities like walking, hiking, or cycling for leisure. Focus on staying active without putting too much strain on muscles.	High
7	Turkey Sausage Breakfast Skillet	Avocado Tuna Boats	Cauliflower Hummus	Steak with Garlic Butter Mushrooms	Strength Training	Repeat full-body strength training routine with an emphasis on progressive overload. Increase weights or intensity for continued muscle growth.	Low
8	Granola Parfait with Yogurt	Black Bean and Corn Salad	Whole Grain Toast with Jam	Quinoa Stuffed Bell Peppers	HIIT Cardio	Perform another HIIT session with different exercises or variations to keep challenging the body. Focus on maximum effort during intervals.	High
9	Almond Flour Pancakes	Egg Salad Lettuce Wraps	Caprese Skewers	Grilled Salmon with Asparagus	Yoga/Pilates	Continue with yoga or Pilates to improve flexibility,	Low

						balance, and core strength. Experiment with new poses or longer holds.	
10	Sweet Potato Hash with Eggs	Veggie Sushi Rolls with Brown Rice	Hummus and Veggie Wrap	Teriyaki Tofu Stir-Fry with Brown Rice	Cardio	Engage in another session of moderate-intensity cardio, such as cycling, rowing, or using an elliptical machine. Maintain a steady pace for endurance.	High
11	Veggie and Cheese Omelet	Greek Salad with Feta and Olives	Cucumber and Cream Cheese Bites	Eggplant Lasagna Roll-Ups	Circuit Training	Switch up the circuit training routine with new exercises and variations. Keep the intensity high to elevate heart rate and burn calories.	Low
12	Blueberry Oat Bran Muffins	Brown Rice and Black Bean Burrito Bowl	Banana Bread	Black Bean Enchiladas with Brown Rice	Active Rest	Enjoy an active rest day with light activities like gardening, gentle stretching, or recreational sports. Focus on relaxation and recovery.	High
13	Coconut Flour Porridge	Cauliflower Fried Rice	Eggplant Chips	Keto Chicken Parmesan	Strength Training	Focus on specific muscle groups with isolation exercises like bicep curls, tricep extensions, and calf raises. Maintain proper form and aim for muscle fatigue.	Low

14	Oatmeal with Fresh Fruit	Pasta Primavera with Whole Wheat Pasta	Baked Sweet Potato Fries	Sweet Potato and Chickpea Buddha Bowl	HIIT Cardio	Perform a challenging HIIT workout incorporating plyometric movements like box jumps, squat jumps, and lateral bounds. Push yourself to the limit.	High
15	Keto Chia Seed Pudding	Grilled Chicken Salad with Avocado	Stuffed Celery Sticks	Greek Lemon Chicken Skewers	Yoga/Pilates	Dedicate this day to deep stretching and relaxation with restorative yoga or Pilates. Focus on breathing and releasing tension in muscles.	Low
16	Fruit Salad with Greek Yogurt	Couscous Salad with Grilled Vegetables	Hummus and Veggie Wrap	Corn and Black Bean Quesadillas	Cardio	Engage in an extended cardio session outdoors such as hiking, running trails, or cycling in nature. Enjoy the scenery and fresh air.	High
17	Zucchini Hash Browns	Zucchini Noodles with Pesto	Cottage Cheese and Tomato Cuts	Spaghetti Squash with Meatballs	Circuit Training	Challenge yourself with an intense circuit incorporating weights or resistance bands. Include exercises like kettlebell swings, resistance band rows, and jump squats.	Low
18	Quinoa Breakfast Bowl	Whole Grain Wrap with Hummus and Veggies	Chocolate Banana Oat Bars	Vegetable Paella	Active Rest	Spend the day participating in recreational activities like swimming, playing tennis, or	High

					dancing. Keep moving and have fun.	
19	Greek Yogurt with Berries	Salmon Cucumber Roll-Ups	Stuffed Mini Bell Peppers	Shrimp and Avocado Salad	Strength Training	Target different muscle groups with a variety of exercises using free weights, machines, or bodyweight. Focus on form and control.	Low
20	Brown Rice Breakfast Bowl	Falafel Pita Sandwich	Banana Bread	Veggie Stir-Fry with Rice Noodles	HIIT Cardio	Try a new HIIT workout format such as Tabata intervals, EMOM (every minute on the minute), or AMRAP (as many rounds as possible) to keep things interesting.	High
21	Almond Flour Pancakes	Spinach and Mushroom Quiche	Caprese Skewers	Chicken and Vegetable Stir-Fry	Yoga/Pilates	Incorporate deep stretching and mobility exercises into your yoga or Pilates routine. Focus on improving range of motion and flexibility.	Low
22	Whole Wheat Pancakes with Maple Syrup	Lentil and Vegetable Stew	Baked Sweet Potato Fries	Vegetarian Chili with Whole Grain Bread	Cardio	Engage in a low-impact cardio activity like swimming or cycling to give your joints a break while still getting a good workout.	High
23	Avocado Egg Salad	Turkey Lettuce Wraps	Eggplant Chips	Chicken Alfredo Zucchini Noodles	Circuit Training	Mix up your circuit routine with different equipment like resistance bands,	Low

					medicine balls, or TRX straps. Keep the intensity high for maximum results.	
24	Blueberry Oat Bran Muffins	Barley and Vegetable Stir-Fry	Fruit and Yogurt Parfait	Chickpea Curry with Basmati Rice	Active Rest	Enjoy a day of active leisure such as playing recreational sports, going for a leisurely bike ride, or taking a long walk in nature.	High
25	Bacon and Egg Muffins	Zucchini Lasagna	Cauliflower Hummus	Taco Stuffed Avocados	Strength Training	Focus on progressive overload by increasing weights or resistance in your strength training routine. Push yourself to lift heavier or perform more reps.	Low
26	Sweet Potato Hash with Eggs	Sweet Potato and Kale Salad	Whole Grain Toast with Jam	Lentil and Vegetable Soup with Whole Grain Bread	HIIT Cardio	Incorporate bodyweight exercises like push-ups, burpees, and mountain climbers into your HIIT routine for a challenging full-body workout.	High
27	Cauliflower Breakfast Hash	Shrimp and Broccoli Stir-Fry	Cucumber and Cream Cheese Bites	Turkey Stuffed Bell Peppers	Yoga/Pilates	Practice mindfulness and relaxation with a gentle yoga or Pilates session focusing on deep breathing and meditation.	Low

28	Quinoa Breakfast Bowl	Chickpea and Spinach Curry	Banana Nut Muffins	Barley Salad with Roasted Vegetables	Cardio	Go for a long-distance run or bike ride to challenge your endurance and cardiovascular fitness. Enjoy the rhythm of your breathing and movement.	High
29	Coconut Flour Porridge	Cauliflower Crust Pizza	Caprese Skewers	Lemon Herb Baked Cod	Circuit Training	Create a circuit using functional movements like squats, lunges, and rows to improve overall strength and coordination. Keep transitions between exercises smooth and efficient.	Low
30	Multigrain Waffles with Honey	Lentil Soup with Whole Grain Bread	Banana Bread	Whole Grain Pizza with Vegetables	Active Rest	Spend time outdoors engaging in low-intensity activities like hiking, walking, or playing frisbee. Focus on enjoying movement without pushing yourself too hard.	High

Conclusion

Congratulations on completing your journey through "The Ultimate Carb Cycling Cookbook for Beginners." This comprehensive guide has equipped you with the knowledge and tools necessary to harness the power of carb cycling to achieve your weight loss and fitness goals effectively. Whether you're looking to shed extra body fat, build lean muscle mass, improve metabolic health, or enhance athletic performance, carb cycling offers a flexible and sustainable approach to nutrition that can be tailored to fit your individual needs and preferences.

Throughout this cookbook and guide, we've explored the fundamentals of carb cycling, including its definition, principles, and benefits. We've delved into the science behind carb cycling and its efficacy for weight loss, providing you with a solid understanding of how and why this approach works. You've learned how to get started with carb cycling, including step-by-step guidance on implementing the strategy, tailoring it to your weight loss goals, and practical advice for success.

As you embark on your carb cycling journey, I encourage you to explore the delicious recipes included in this book and experiment with different meal combinations to keep your meals interesting and satisfying. From hearty breakfasts to flavorful dinners and nutritious snacks, you'll find a variety of options to suit your tastes and preferences.

If you found "The Ultimate Carb Cycling Cookbook for Beginners" helpful and informative, I invite you to leave a positive review and share your feedback with others. Your reviews and testimonials not only help me improve as an author but also inspire and motivate others to embark on their own journey towards better health and wellness. Together, we can make a positive impact and empower individuals around the world to live their best lives.

Thank you for choosing "The Ultimate Carb Cycling Cookbook for Beginners." Here's to your success and a healthier, fitter you!

Printed in Great Britain
by Amazon